PRAISE
WILD WORLD, J

"*Wild World, Joyful Heart* is an important book—and a timely companion—when so many are suffering and wondering how to bring more health and joy into their lives. Laurie Warren delivers both intriguing philosophy and tactical steps in this enjoyable and easy read. She writes in a way that will draw you in and leave you with unshakeable confidence on how to feel better in your everyday life."

—Emma Seppälä, PhD, Stanford and Yale professor
and author of *The Happiness Track*

"The essence of *Wild World, Joyful Heart* is empowerment. Laurie Warren masterfully explores the science and philosophy behind why we stay stuck in our unhealthy and unhappy existence—and provides the keys to turn that paradigm around. Her compassion, humor, and actionable steps will have you dancing to a whole new beat of health and joy."

—Mark C. Perna, author of the award-winning bestseller,
Answering Why; keynote speaker; and CEO

"Laurie Warren's debut wellness book, *Wild World, Joyful Heart*, is a tour de force. With passion and compassion, the author explores our relationship with mind, body, and spirit, both individually and collectively. She offers hard-won wisdom drawn from her own life experiences to guide readers toward greater self-knowledge and self-care and, ultimately, toward embracing personal and societal responsibility. We live in challenging times. Laurie contributes not just new insights, seamlessly woven together, but practical guidance for thriving amidst the chaos."

—Deborah Sosin, LICSW, author of *Charlotte and the Quiet Place*
and *Breaking Free of Addiction*

"Laurie Warren leads us on a journey toward wholeness by helping us realize our own untapped potential and reminding us of the important connection between joy and hardship."

—Lindsay Tucker, *Yoga Journal*

"Laurie Warren's *Wild World, Joyful Heart* fills me with a redefined sense of commitment. As the founder of Beyond Mom, a community committed to greater fulfillment for women and mothers, I recognize we're living in a complicated time in history: There's greater stress caused by world affairs, technology domination, fast-paced schedules, and a culture that tells us we should be perfect; our health and well-being are suffering. Laurie's book reminds me that there is a trail being blazed by light workers who have the tools to decrease stress, increase self-care and self-awareness, and achieve perspective in a world that too often overwhelms us. All parts of ourselves: body, mind, and energy must be nurtured and upheld to their optimum potential. Laurie, thank you for writing this book and providing a compass for so many."

—Randi Zinn, author of *Going Beyond Mom: How to Activate Your Mind, Body, & Business after Baby*

WILD WORLD, JOYFUL HEART

LAURIE WARREN

WILD WORLD, JOYFUL HEART

UNLOCK YOUR POWER
TO CREATE HEALTH AND JOY

To Jess,
and your
health & joy

—

RIVER GROVE
BOOKS

Published by River Grove Books
Austin, TX
www.rivergrovebooks.com

Distributed by River Grove Books

Design and composition by Greenleaf Book Group and Brian Phillips
Cover design by Greenleaf Book Group and Brian Phillips

Publisher's Cataloging-in-Publication data is available.

Print ISBN: 978-1-63299-247-5

eBook ISBN: 978-1-63299-248-2

First Edition

For Nunu.
And, for my four loves: Alex, Carolyn, Connor, and Jen.

CONTENTS

FOREWORD

Sitting in my home in British Columbia looking out over the Pacific Ocean sharing a coffee with a dear friend, I was deep in angst over a personal issue. I was stuck in my experience of emotional pain. My friend reminded me to shift my eyes 2 inches to the left and connect to what I see. "It is stunningly beautiful," I said. He reminded me that our feelings are often a product of where we put our eyes; beauty and pain often exist at the same time.

Wild World, Joyful Heart brings to light this understanding of the dichotomous journey of the human condition, simultaneously connecting us to joy and challenge. This deceptively breezy title tackles deep and philosophical ideas offering wisdom, experience, and knowledge from a wealth of differing sources. Who are we? How can we embody our best selves? What is our relationship to one another and to the universe in which we inhabit? Journeying through these pages, guidance is offered supporting the "evolution of self" as a component of healing our torn planet, "stitching up our wounded world." Beginning with theory and moving into practical applications, *Wild World, Joyful Heart* emphasizes the development of a healthier body, mind, and connection to spirit.

I have known Laurie Warren for over a decade. She is a change agent—a brave, brilliant, and insightful paradigm pioneer. As a mental health occupational therapist, I have referred clients to Laurie primarily for her expertise as a holistic nutritionist, but also knowing that she blends knowledge from a multitude of disciplines with compassion and with care. Laurie is very curious, a spiritual wayfarer, and passionate about helping people to be their best selves. Her book represents all of these qualities, and her quirky and unique communication style makes the concepts understandable and relatable. Her descriptions of how emotions, stress, and trauma interact support the reader in beginning to appreciate that our potential to transform is truly within our capacity. As anyone with curiosity knows, life is full of wonder. *Wild World, Joyful Heart* is an insightful exploration of all these ups and downs—a celebration of what can be.

—**KIM BARTHEL, OT**
Co-author of *Conversations with a Rattlesnake*

OUT OF THE GATE: PROMISE, BIRTH, AND INVITATION

Standing on the Edge of Fantastic Promise

"I wish I felt better. More happy and healthy."

The majority of our population has this thought daily. We struggle with physical challenges like our weight, disease and illness, and lack of energy. We struggle with mental challenges like stress, addiction, emotional drama, a poor self-image, and loneliness. We wonder: *What's wrong with me?* or *What does this all mean, anyway?*

I've been thinking about helping people unlock their potential for health and joy for a long time. From a young age, I've had a love affair with the living world and everything in it, most especially people. This love affair unfolded gradually, fueled at first by curiosity, then increasingly passion. It led me, eventually, to work that guides people toward more health and joy—toward becoming the most vibrant version of themselves that they're ready to embody. What's also apparent, from my work and from living at this moment, is that modern humanity stands at a critical tipping point between peril and promise.

Yes, our modern world can feel scary. Thanks to our 24/7 cable news culture, we have a constant view into increasing levels of political unrest, chronic disease, obesity, poverty, violence, addiction, thirst, and hunger, all amid a rapid population growth across the globe. With that as our life soundtrack, it's natural to feel confused or afraid. *What's happening?! Why do others seem to have so much, while I work so hard and have so little? Why do I feel tired, unhealthy, lonely, anxious, and dissatisfied?*

What we really want is to *feel different,* in our everyday life experience. The great news is that you're not alone, and this is not the end of the story.

These very concerns that many of us are grappling with—the perils and challenges that plague us individually and globally—are exactly why we're living on the edge of fantastic promise, individually and as a species. History teaches us that groundbreaking change is made in response to peril and painful challenges. A wild world can actually generate joyful hearts. We're navigating an increasingly complex environment—social, political, technological, scientific, religious, spiritual, commercial, and informational—that is changing more rapidly than at any prior time in our evolution as a species. With things moving so fast, it's easy to get caught up in the speed and in the doing—to lose our grounding connection to our sense of self, to our well-being, and to our connection to everything around us.

But we have the power to change this. *Our mind is either the bridge or the barrier to everything we want physically, emotionally, relationally, and spiritually.* We possess the power to heal, to use our astounding creative powers, to realize self-trust and personal clarity, and to connect—with self, with other, and with something a lot bigger—in a way that brings satisfaction and meaning to our everyday existence.

How might that feel? Imagine waking up with energy and feeling ready for your day. You dress a healthy body that you feel comfortable inhabiting. Your mind is clear and focused as you move through your day, and you're largely unfettered by stress or emotional drama. Problems and difficulties invariably crop up, and your response to them is rational and solution-oriented. You enjoy strong, supportive relationships and know how to weather their expected challenges. You feel connected to those around you, connected to the deepest part of yourself, and accepting of who you are. You would feel, for the most part, content with your life experience. We possess this healthy and joyful life experience in its potentiated state—every single one of us.

I've worked for decades as a change agent for health, joy, and personal evolution—guiding people toward a fuller expression of their potential. This work is my passion and my joy. Between the covers of this book, you'll find an integrated buffet of the philosophy and tools that I share with my clients and students. We'll explore the myths in our wild world that keep you stuck in dis-ease and discontent. You'll learn about the power of habits and how to put them to work for you, instead of against you. We'll tour the three foundational pillars of personal responsibility, self-worth, and self-care and then we'll follow with theory and on-the-ground tactics on how to honor your body, tend your mind, and live your spirit. Lastly, we'll delve into how all that potentiated YOU can positively resonate out to your relationships and the world around you. The world that we all share. I wrote this book for you, and for all of us—the whole human family.

A Book Is Born

Speaking of family, I talk to my mom every day. Judy Warren is a loving mother, an independent thinker, a talented artist, an ardent gardener and nature enthusiast, a survivor, and an eighty-seven-year-old wise and grounded sage. She's fun and funny, and she's one of my best friends. Recently, I was talking to her about my work on this book and she said, "I can't wait to read it. I hope it doesn't have one of those horrible long introductions—those are so boring." I chuckled and said, "Well, the great thing about the introduction, Mom, is that you can skip it and still receive all that the author wants to share with you. . . . And, Mom? You're gonna want to skip the introduction in my book. It's long."

We had a good laugh. You see, when I read a book, I'm quite interested in the being who wrote it. Knowing them, on some level, helps ground me in their ideas. It provides me with some background and context for the insights and information that the author felt moved to share. Please don't feel obliged to read this introduction just because it's in front of you. However, if, like me, you're interested in getting acquainted with an author's becoming, as well as their reasons for birthing a book, then by all means, read on. Happily for you, I'll circumnavigate the bulk of the first three decades of my life.

The year I turned thirty was the year I became a woman—a full-fledged adult. Four events transpired over the final three months of 1996 that escorted me out of the self-absorption that often presides over our twenties, and into a more expanded and selfless approach to life. I got married, became a stepmother to two amazing young girls, left the career I'd been working hard to build, and, almost overnight, my brother-in-law Buz succumbed to cancer. He was only forty-seven years old and had been like a big brother since I was fourteen. I was an "oops" baby, with my two sisters being nine and eleven years older than me, so I was fortunate to acquire two beloved brothers (in-law) during my teen years.

As I mentioned earlier, groundbreaking change is most often made in response to peril and painful challenge; this is true globally and personally. The year 1996 offered me some personal experience with this truth. Buz's abrupt exit found me ill-equipped to work through my grief, and my heart ached for my sister. Alongside this, I was filled with love for my husband and stepdaughters, while also feeling unsure in my new role as a stepparent; and I was challenged by the turbulent waters of my husband's relationship with his ex-wife.

On the professional front, I knew I didn't want the career as a finance manager in high tech that I had worked so hard to build, but I wasn't sure what I did want. Times of personal challenge can often be aided by therapy, and the psychologist I'd been seeing for career counseling was now also serving me as a grief counselor and a stepmom counselor.

I am a great lover of books and have been an avid reader and learning junkie since my youth. I began reading philosophy, psychology, health, and self-help books in my late teens. So it's fitting that it was a book that changed my course in 1996. Buz was diagnosed with a large and aggressive brain tumor in April of that year, and he and my sister Linda were utilizing a wide variety of conventional and alternative approaches to eradicate the cancer cells and encourage his body to heal. One day when visiting their cabin on the coast of Maine, I saw a book on the kitchen table called *Beating Cancer with Nutrition* by Patrick Quillin, PhD. I wondered, what on earth did food have to do with disease? I leafed through it, was captivated, and bought my own copy upon returning home to Massachusetts.

I finished reading the book in a day, complete with my usual highlights and margin notes. I felt something in me shift, as I resonated with the science and the author's healing approach in the book, which also aligned with what I'd learned firsthand over the preceding months. From Elaine, my therapist, I'd learned about human uniqueness and that we have a choice in how we think about things. From Quillin's book, I'd taken away that we build our body, every day, with food. Not just fill our stomach or even fuel our body, but literally *build* or construct our body. (This doesn't mean that Buz necessarily built his cancer with food. Although food—type, quality, and quantity—is often a contributing factor to all disease, becoming unwell can be more complicated than that.) The fire had been lit. I was hungry for awareness and healing, for myself and for those around me. I didn't know it at the time, but the fulcrum was now in place on which the rest of my life would turn.

I did continue working in high tech for another four years, now in sales, as I was still loosely enjoying the constant learning, creating, and pivoting that this sector requires. However, I had also become fascinated with what makes us well and what makes us unwell—in our bodies and minds.

The next dozen years found me stepparenting my girls and parenting the boys I gave birth to in my mid-thirties. I was a working mom and then a stay-at-home mom and then a volunteer health-worker mom. I was interested with how food affects the body and began experimenting with healthy eating myself and with my family.

And I studied obsessively—fascinated with the body, the mind, and, increasingly, with spirit. I got involved with an international nutrition foundation and began lecturing around the Boston area. I took courses when my parenting responsibilities allowed, following my passion to learn about health, psychology, mindfulness, and ancient wisdom. The autumn that my sons entered full-day elementary school, I enrolled in graduate school. Two years later, I earned a master's degree in clinical and integrative nutrition and started my own wellness company.

In the few years after opening my company, I was launched into what I affectionately call my "Midlife Awakening." I've never been a fan of the term *midlife crisis* because it implies that something bad is happening. What happens for many of us in midlife can—if approached with curiosity, humility, and openness—become a time of intense and meaningful change. Of personal evolution.

On the professional front, I completed additional training in functional medicine and herbalism and began using lab work in my clinical and integrative health practice, specializing in digestion, endocrinology, and cancer. My work also expanded to include corporate work, helping companies build progressive wellness cultures.

On the personal front, my marriage had become increasingly strained and disconnected. I loved my husband and he was an excellent man, but our communication issues had worsened; I felt an important thread had been broken beyond repair—and this really knocked me on my ass. We divorced in 2013. We mustered up the most mindful and respectful divorce we could, but it was still messy and painful. It launched me further into self-inquiry, growth, and expansion, which has continued as I've grown my business and single/co-parented in the years since. Those Midlife Awakening years also launched me into new areas of study and training, including subtle systems and energy healing, Mindfulness-Based Stress Reduction (MBSR), immunology, and genetics. Over the years, I've become equally fascinated with science and spirituality and have come to understand that they have much more in common than is typically thought. The hook for me is that they both, in their pure state, seek to understand the natural world in order to support life and understanding.

We, as a species, know surprisingly little. Yes, after my half-century school-of-life training—that saw me try five careers and seven jobs, go through seven years of college, psychotherapy, hundreds of nonfiction books and research studies, marriage and divorce—I'm continually awed by how little the human species knows about itself and its environment. I also learned that formal schooling is partly about learning what *other* people think and then accepting that as fact. This isn't always instructive, nor does it do much for creative thinking. I believe it's more important to develop curiosity, to discover *how* to think; and I would argue that's when real learning and understanding begins. The majority of what has fed my expertise and wisdom, I learned outside of a formal classroom.

In the end, I think the most important thing about a person is how we move through the world, how we relate to ourselves and others, and how we synthesize and assimilate the lessons and wisdom that are ripe for harvest in everyday life. Our co-creators—the folks alongside whom we learn and grow—are also important contributors to our understanding and growth.

I've had fifty-plus years of ongoing connections, conversations, and professional collaboration with people who shape who I'm continually becoming. We humans are the complex fabric of who we are, what and who we've experienced, and how we've put that all together. How do we assimilate and apply what we learn? For me, my drive for understanding is about two questions:

1. How can we set ourselves up to realize our untapped potential—to thrive in body and mind, and to more fully express our spirit?

2. How can our thriving as potentiated individuals contribute to solving our global challenges?

Hence, I gave birth to this book, which combines personal experiential reflections with findings from my clinical and integrative health practice, alongside my interdisciplinary studies in science, psychology, and spirituality. The common draw that these disciplines of science, psychology, and spirituality hold for me is that they can all be used to support the thriving human organism living on a healthy, integrated planet. As an eternally curious person, the fact that there's so much that we don't understand in these disciplines attracts me.

The fields within these disciplines that I draw on—biology, biochemistry, neuroscience, functional medicine, philosophy, psychology, wisdom traditions, and more—have been around for many years. What I offer to you is a unique synthesis of these fields along with recent compelling scientific discoveries, provided alongside what has worked best for my clients and students for decades.

In a sense, this is a book of themes—a book of powerful beginnings. Not only could each chapter become its own book, but each section within each chapter could become its own book. This means that the intent is not one of exhaustive exploration of each topic but instead a juicy, fleshed-out summary of what's important in your journey toward health and joy.

The philosophy, information, and stories that follow are presented in a logical order; however, they can also be read in disordered chunks that you absorb and work with. At heart, I'm a fun-loving person who likes to laugh and goof around, and I tire of rigidity quickly. Thus, in addition to a healthy dose of science, psychology, and philosophy in the following pages, you'll also find colloquial prose and some goofy humor.

You'll further find, in a few key places, questions that have come from my clients and students over the years. They're questions that I often get asked in response to the ideas presented here. These questions are presented in italics and are separated from the body of the text. I included them because sometimes, when taking in new information, we feel questions that we can't quite put into words yet—they're more of a niggling feeling. My hope is that these questions, and their answers, contribute to the ease of your journey through this book.

You hold in your hands the book I wish I'd had when I was twenty-six. This is a book for everyday people like you and me who want to live a good life in a more sane world. This book was born to empower you to create the life experience you desire. This book isn't about changing who you are. It's about changing your experience to bring you contentment. Where you choose to consciously evolve because you want to be more joyful, not because there's anything wrong with you. This book is about love. Love for self, love for others, and reverence for all the millions of ways that love has manifested on this planet. This book is about personal evolution toward health, joy, and wholeness.

An Invitation

How do we manifest our potential for health and joy? We'll be getting to that in the next eleven chapters, but first let's get clear on exactly what we're talking about here. Throughout your exploration of this book, I will use terms that may not be familiar to you or that I explain because I want to be crystal clear about what I mean when using them. These words will be in bold when I first use them and followed by an explanation. They're also included in a glossary in the back of the book for quick and easy reference, so when they come up again later, you can easily refresh your memory. I bring this up now because I want to be clear about the words that you read in the subtitle: Unlock Your Power to Create Health and Joy. Health and joy are what this book is about, so let's get on the same page as to what, exactly, we're creating.

Health is balance, integration, and ease—overall well-being—in body, emotions, mind, and spirit. This is whole-person health that we create from within and nurture on an ongoing basis. The idea of health is simple, in concept, whereas many people are confused about joy. **Joy** is different from happiness. Happiness is a good feeling, and it's also dependent on outside circumstances—a transient and fickle visitor. If you give me a bowl of ice cream, I feel happy; if you take it away, I don't feel happy anymore. Joy is an attitude that arises from the heart and spirit and is not affected by outside circumstances. Joy, in a very real way, is experiencing exactly what's happening, minus our opinion of it. Hence, it's possible to feel joy when someone takes away our ice cream, or during challenging times. Joy is connected to our inner peace, to our acceptance of the present moment, and to our awareness of connection—to one another, to life itself, and to something larger than ourselves. This is why this book is not about health and happiness. Most of us, although we may not have thought about it, are hankering for joy, because life is hard and happiness cannot be depended upon. Joy can.

You can take the first step toward health and joy right here, right now, by simply embracing the idea that health and joy are a journey. Journeys are less about the destination and more about what happens along the way. You are a unique and exquisite person with every right to be here learning, exploring, and creating. A journey of continually judging yourself as good or bad, healthy or unhealthy, deserving or undeserving, joyful or miserable—is a journey of missing the point. You're a creator and a decision-maker living in a world of possibilities and probabilities. Each moment of your life provides you with the opportunity to move closer to the fullness of who you are, or further away. Closer to health and joy, or further away. In the end, only you know the difference. Judgment means nothing. The journey is everything.

What's essential to the journey of personal evolution—to change—is not information, but *understanding.* In the digital age, a person can have information about many things and at the same time understand nothing at all. Oh, but understanding is ooh-la-la! Understanding is different from education or information. It can include the synthesis of those things, but it's so much more. Understanding is a creative process that can be attained only by personal creative synthesis and application, then back to personal creative synthesis, and on to application again, and so on.

This continual process is what begets understanding. Cognitively grasping an idea is only the seed—a kick-ass and important seed, but still a seed.

It's our intentional, iterative understanding and living of an idea that gives it meaning and that unlocks our potential for the health and joy that reside within us. Ansel Adams, landscape photographer and environmentalist, said, "In wisdom gathered over time, I have found that every experience is a form of exploration." How fun! We're on an exploration together, a journey, an adventure. We've invited each other into the adventure that is *you*.

Yes, picking up this book means you're inviting me to contribute to your journey toward wholeness—healthy body, calm and steady mind, joy, and personal evolution. Please know that I don't take that invitation lightly. The reader experience that I invite you to consider involves taking in what you read with an open heart and mind. Not in honor of me or of this book, but in honor of you and your journey. Hence, this book is not a suggestion of one particular way to live a joyful and healthy life. I've worked with enough clients and struggled with enough of my own health issues over the years—IBS, pre-diabetes, Lyme disease, food sensitivities, a challenging menopause transition, and chronic myalgia—to know that health is not linear and healing is not a one-size-fits-all answer. This book is not prescriptive in the sense of a rigid protocol; instead, it is an invitation.

I invite you to the ideas in this book in the same way that someone is invited to a dance. (I absolutely love dancing, so this is one heartfelt invitation.) This is not an invitation to be all serious and thinking that you have so much to "fix" about yourself. For ha-has, let's say you did every single thing in this book—then what? The truth is, there is no destination and no perfect you. Instead, the truth is the everyday exploration, contemplation, and learning—a leaning in, if you will—that's the journey. I invite you to frolic through the pages of this book and to do things that are delightful to you. I invite you to join the dance by embracing the moves that resonate with you and leaving the ones that don't for another dancer.

In this way, this book becomes your unique dance. I encourage you to highlight in it, doodle funny faces in it, write notes in it about what *you* think. Create a personalized handbook that becomes your own personal philosophy and approach to fully engaging with your evolution—and your glorious path toward a more vibrant life experience. I also invite you to consider your resonance with what you read. The point isn't to force your experience to match something you read. This book is a guide for working with and understanding your experience, in whatever form that takes. There's no right or wrong here. No mandated goals or shoulds. At the end of each chapter, I invite you to ask yourself: What in there resonated for me?

I also invite you to embrace that you're enough right now, that your aspirations and intentions for a new way of experiencing life are attainable, *and* that your aspirations for a new way of experiencing life are completely congruent with being enough right now. *How can this be?* It's a case of "Yes And." *Yes*, you are enough; *and* our purpose on this planet is to learn, grow, create, and evolve. Not because we "should," but because it's awesome and fun and healthy, and it helps us feel vibrantly alive. To become ever more of who we truly are. A rosebud is perfect and is incredibly beautiful. It's enough, just as it is; and every rosebud aspires to become a rose flower—to bloom into more of itself. We're all like that rose, even if we haven't fully woken up to it yet. Wake up to it, we must—for ourselves, and for our wild and crazy world.

Healed people heal people. My small act of writing a book is both for individuals and for the global collective. I know that's a big wish. Remember, though, everything starts small. And I believe we're evolving to a new way of being that isn't compromised by chronic poor physical health, closed and polarized by the untended mind, twisted by our emotions, stuck in fear, or disconnected from spirit. We'll increasingly nourish our body, tend our mind, and align with our spirit while living the most authentic, connected, and loving version of ourselves, as our sum becomes exponentially more than its parts. We will integrate body, mind, and spirit to enrich our experience— both personally and globally.

Thank you for inviting me to share what I've learned with you. My hope is that, somewhere in these pages, you'll recognize yourself in all your innate wholeness and uniquely scrumptious imperfection—and that you'll accept my invitation to join our conscious evolution toward better health and more joy.

CHAPTER 1

WILD WORLD

"All I know is, I just feel—unhappy. It's not just the extra forty-five pounds, although that's part of it. I'm so stressed out—it's like I'm always running against time. And the news is depressing—it's like the world's falling apart. Honestly? I feel starved for everything healthy and real and good."

Meet Kate. She's your average, middle-aged, middle-class working parent—an attractive, delightfully edgy, plump woman who lives a relatively comfortable life. She eats when she wants to and has a warm place to lay her head at night. She also has a job, two kids, and goes on vacation once a year. I met Kate at a networking event and she later became a client. (An interesting aspect of the work I do is that even fleeting discussions with a new acquaintance can quickly veer toward the deep and personal.)

I've heard Kate's sentiment expressed by clients, friends, and relatives many times, in countless ways. People are struggling—with their weight, with chronic health issues, stress and fatigue, life balance, and with feeling as if they're on a hamster wheel. They're wondering why there's this niggling feeling of emptiness and loneliness, of unsatisfactoriness, of what-does-it-all-mean-anyway? The craziness, the political unrest, and the polarization of the world around them only add fuel to the fire. Similar to Kate, people have a lot of worry about the world, but feel like a spectator watching their world spin into deeper dysfunction. That's a lot to unpack, and that's exactly what we're going to do as we explore the ideas in this book.

Before we get into the juicy, empowering chapters to come, let's peek under the covers at some of what might be getting in the way of your living your best life. What are some of the key cultural factors that are informing your life experience? These hidden factors clandestinely affect your everyday choices, decisions, and life experience, and they aren't your fault. Meaning, you didn't create them, but you do have the ability to override them, and that's exactly what Chapters 2 through 11 (the rest of the book) are about.

These factors, because they're off our radar, typically lead us to internalize their negative power and blame ourselves when we don't feel good in our life experience. All that needless blame holds us back even more, sending us into a downward spiral, like Kate. And that's not the direction we want our spiral to go. We want spirals of evolution, not devolution. We want vibrant health and joy, not poor health and unhappiness. These first two chapters are about the ways you can let yourself off the hook and move forward in full, glorious ownership of your life experience—creating health and joy. And we're going to start with the world-view of a fish, as we prepare to take a tour through some common cultural myths that hold us back from our potential.

If a fish is swimming around in the ocean and a scuba diver appears in front of her and says, "Wow! Look at all this water you live in. It seems to go on forever, in every direction," the fish would say, "Huh? What's 'water'?" *Because* it's surrounding her, the fish isn't aware of the very water she's spent her entire life in.

This same phenomenon happens with people—like Kate and like many of us—except the water that we swim in is our culture. When experiences and data repeat themselves, they become familiar, and our mind labels them as normal—and, often, as trusted. When the repeated experience is something like well-maintained roads that we get to drive our car on, seeing that as normal is a good thing. When the repeated experience is weight gain, chronic fatigue, stress, disease, neglect, marginalization, or some other form of imbalance, coming to see it as normal is not a good thing. Common and normal are not the same thing.

The following modern-day myths that contribute to our wild world are all examples of common-but-not-normal, and they are the water in which we swim. Each of these contributing cultural aspects have become ubiquitous in our daily life experience. They are so widely accepted as normal that we simply don't see how they keep us from unlocking our potential to be healthy and joyful. We're that proverbial fish that can't see the water they're swimming in. *"What water? What the heck is water?!"*

Myth: Popular Equals Good/Right

"Everything popular is wrong," wrote Oscar Wilde. I think one of the biggest mistakes we make in our life experience is to confuse popularity with "rightness." We confuse what's common with what's normal. It's easy to confuse common and normal, so we tend to slowly recalibrate our thinking to accommodate what's common, even if it doesn't feel good, so that we feel normal. Then, we don't notice it much anymore—it's just the way it is. By accepting it as "the way it is," we feel the camaraderie and connection of our shared suffering—but this doesn't help us feel, or live, better.

It's important that we notice and become discerning about what we accept into our lives—because our life experience is shaped by what we surround ourselves with, and by what we buy into. Our life experience is shaped by the intersection of our minds with our environments. We often fall into the trap of accepting something into the fabric of our precious life experience without noticing how it feels for us. For instance, how do I feel as a result of watching the news before bed? Do I feel light or heavy, content or fearful, relaxed or anxious? The fact is, the culture we live in causes us pain, but this pain itself is so common that we lose sight of the fact that it's not normal.

Myth: Human as Machine

In recent decades, our culture has become more open to discussions about body, mind, and spirit. Yet many folks still talk about these three aspects as if they're separate, as with hammer, nail, and lumber. These three aspects of a construction project are completely separate material things; however, body, mind, and spirit are not. Almost anything we do in one aspect of our humanity affects the other aspects. Further, within each of those aspects, there is deep interconnectedness. For instance, if I take a medication to suppress my cholesterol production, this has far-reaching effects in all of my body, not simply in cholesterol production. If I eat a lot of sugar, it's going to affect many interconnected systems and organs in my body; it will also affect my brain (which is part of the body, although most people don't think of it that way).

Our current medical/health insurance/pharmaceutical paradigm is to approach each part of our body as if it were an island unto itself. We have doctors for many separate body parts—heart doctor (several types), brain doctor (several types), reproductive doctor, lung doctor, digestive doctor— as if we were human machines with independently operating body parts and systems. We even consider some of our parts dispensable: our adenoids, gall bladder, pieces of our stomach, and sections of our intestine. We also send "prescribed" chemicals (pharmaceutical drugs) into our interconnected parts without questioning how they'll affect the body's overall environment. We don't think about what other parts these chemicals are interfering with, or how these chemicals interact *with each other*. Or, how they interact with the pesticides in our food. I've worked with countless people who are living the unpleasant aftermath of this human-as-machine approach.

Myth: We're Alone in Our Struggles

A truth that has become apparent over the years of my work with individuals and groups is that which is the most personal is also the most universal. This is an idea originally attributed to renowned psychologist Carl R. Rogers. In other words, we feel as if we have some unique private corner on our specific pain, neurosis, relationship issues, health problems, addiction, checkered past, emotional eating, social drama, parenting blunders, work challenges, and life-balance struggles. But in reality, our struggles are quite similar, in the same way that vanilla and strawberry ice cream are made of the same basic ingredients, with a variation in flavorings. I tell you this not to communicate that you're un-special, but to shine a light on the support, connection, and healing that's available, if only we open to it.

The trouble is, to lean into that support, connection, and healing, we need to be brave enough to communicate how we're feeling, rather than trying to make everything in our lives look shiny and happy. We need to be brave enough to have our insides and outsides become coherent. We miss out on the common ground available to us because our hyper-connected world isn't necessarily connecting around the ideas that will guide us, heal us, and support self-coherence. This life-saving, healing connection isn't happening because we're busy comparing our insides (in all their messy, flawed detail) to other people's outsides (shiny social media-worthy highlights) and deducing that we're alone.

Client: "I want to lose weight and have more energy, but I really struggle with emotional eating, especially at night. Nothing helps."

Me: "Me too! It's hard, isn't it?"

Client: "Wait. You struggle with emotional eating?" (This said in a tone that would also have accompanied, "Wait. You turn into a werewolf at night?")

Me: "Absolutely. Some days more than others. Our subconscious mind is a slippery bugger! Let's focus on progress instead of perfection and talk about some ideas and tools that can help."

I have this type of conversation with people often—clients, students, friends, family, colleagues—about their health issues and challenges in parenting, loving, and living in the twenty-first century. People often have this idea that I have it all figured out; I must live this charmed life of health, low stress, ease in relationships, and harmonious bliss. In actuality, I *understand* how to unlock my potential, but living it is more of an eternal practice. We must let go of this idea that we struggle while everyone else is living a charmed life. This myth of the insularity of our pain keeps us disconnected, out of balance, and unhappy. What connects us? What are the bridges? From a young age, I've been all about noticing bridges. I can tell you, unequivocally, that our sameness is far, far greater than any of the piddly stuff that separates us—including our struggles.

Myth: Power Equals Truth

There are many powerful forces that shape our culture. A comprehensive exploration of these forces is too much to pursue in these pages and frankly could get a bit doom-and-gloom-ish. I would love for our precious time together to be focused on unlocking your exquisite potential, as opposed to an exhaustive hashing through of the many influences that lead folks to feel the way Kate does. That said, there are a few powerful influences that warrant a shout-out. Our belief in these myths keeps us unempowered, which in turn keeps us from our living our best life experience. These powerful influencers are fear, technology, media, our broken healthcare system, and cultural dogma.

Fear Factor

Fear is everywhere. It's in our news, media, schools, marketing, social media, churches, workplaces, and homes. It affects our daily lives in big and little ways. We're continually hearing our world isn't safe, that people are awful, that we don't have enough, that *we're* not enough. The scarcity- and fear-based messaging that permeates our culture is stealing our health, connections, feelings of wholeness, and our sanity.

One reason that fear is so powerful is that our primal brain (the amygdala) is wired to search the environment for threat and to respond to fear. This hard-wired survival instinct of fear was helpful when we were cavepeople scavenging around looking for berries and instead came across a snarling cave hyena. However, most of our fear today is psychological fear—of things that *might* happen—and there's not much we can do about our worries in the moment. Yet, we still respond to these psychological fears instinctually and with a lot of energy due to hundreds of thousands of years of programming. As a result, many organizations and groups use fear to control us and drive our desires. Our everyday unfounded fears are robbing us of joy, as individuals and as a species.

Technology Trap

We live in an age of rapidly changing digital technology, and it has a powerful influence on our lives. Personal technology, like most things, has a positive side and a negative one. It's helpful, in many ways, to carry a computer around in our pocket or on our wrist. However, this technology that we love and rely on is also silently eroding our self-worth and our connection.

For thousands of years, people have had the internal instinct to create their own self-validation, which assists in creating healthy self-worth. Now, we're becoming dangerously dependent on instant and outside validation, most notably through social media. This feel-good validation lights up the same reward centers in our brain that cocaine, sugar, and heroin do—the dopamine circuit. Outside validation is addictive, and we start to depend on it more and more, until we actually wither without it. Worse, it's not limited to only social media or how many friends, followers, and likes we have. It's also present in email, tweets, texts, snaps, alerts, chats—all of the ways our personal technology devices help us to feel needed or validated by others. This trend, from an evolutionary standpoint, has spread like wildfire, quickly becoming deeply encoded in our habits and social norms. We'll explore this idea more in Chapter 4.

Twisted Triad

I'm certainly not the first one to say that healthcare in America is an expensive, largely ineffective, snarled-up mess. The medical, health insurance, and pharmaceutical industries have interlocked to create a powerful, albeit dysfunctional, monopoly on our state of (poor) health. They amount, in many ways, to sickness-management insurance as opposed to a healthcare system, and we wind up spending a staggering amount of money to simply manage symptoms. Am I fortunate to have a health carrier that pays for some of my medical costs? Yes. Am I happy that pharmaceutical companies make antibiotics when I've got raging bacterial pneumonia? Absolutely. If I were in a car accident or mauled by a rabid coyote, would I be grateful for medical intervention? Damn straight. Because physical health *trauma* is where our medical technology *shines*.

The trouble is, chronic illness is largely what we suffer from. Unfortunately, our healthcare system is not set up to supply adequate or effective care for chronic illness, in support of whole-person health. And the person with chronic illness in the body—the human who has a subjective core of mind and spirit at the heart of their lives—is often discounted. These folks often find their way to my practice. They've shuffled from doctor to doctor and haven't received the time or foundational, whole-person expertise that is required to ignite the healing response. We spent $3.5 *trillion* on US healthcare costs in 2017. This large, deficit-causing expenditure was largely used to manage symptoms, as opposed to educating and healing the whole-person.

We are not empowered in the care of our health. The current patient system is chock-full of folks who are blindly following advice to mask symptoms, while the underlying dysfunction is continuing to manifest and to affect other systems of the body. The medical system is increasingly full of doctors who are struggling with stress-related illness and/or burnout themselves, while the way they practice medicine falls further and further under the control of the pharmaceutical and insurance companies. There is a saying: "There's no money in healthy people or dead people, only in sick people." This is fundamentally true, and medical, health insurance, and pharmaceutical entities are businesses. Businesses seek to make money. Considering how the twisted triad of "sickness management" might be holding you back from your full physical health potential is an important step in reclaiming all of your whole-health potential.

Dogma Downer: Anything Can Become a Religion

The development of dogma turbo-charges the power of the three influences we've just discussed. **Dogma** is when something that starts out as an idea gains traction, and then people start to talk about the idea like it's a 100 percent truth that can't be argued. This is, indeed, what tends to happen in religion, which is why the term *religious dogma* exists: my way is the only right way, the truth. It's important to understand that dogma is not restricted to religion.

Anytime a powerful entity starts to present its ideas as incontrovertible truth, this is dogma. This can happen in religion, yes, but also anywhere else: medicine, science, nutrition, philosophy, politics, economics, scholastics, and so on. As a science lover, I cringe when science is presented as fact. What is cutting-edge science one day sometimes becomes disproven years later. Further, as sociologist William Bruce Cameron wrote, "Not everything that can be counted counts, and not everything that counts can be counted."

It's important to understand that substantial corroboration is all science can really offer—a scientific theory can't be proven as indisputable truth in the way that a math theory can. However, it's most often presented as such, taking on the cloak of dogma.

Dogma takes hold when we stop questioning—when we stop being curious about the information we're taking in. It's been said that if a lie is repeated often enough, it's accepted as truth.

The most important thing to have is an open, curious mind—of understanding that we don't know what we don't know, rather than relying on dogma. From the place of an open mind, we can take in information—people/articles/news shows/books stating things as fact, or when a larger idea is reduced to a flimsy sound bite, or when we hear these things over and over—and remain curious about what's true. Dogma doesn't serve us. Curiosity does. Open-mindedness does. Asking good questions does. Appreciating mystery does. Dogma usually has more to do with keeping power where it's already gathered, and that may not always be a good thing for the rest of us.

Myth: We're Hapless Victims

The cultural water we swim in gives rise to the prevailing belief that our life experience happens *to* us and is dictated by forces outside of our control. We fall into the belief that our despair and happiness come from external people and events. When our body dysfunctions, we blame genetics and we look to doctors and other practitioners to "fix" us. When our relationship goes sour, we blame the other person. When we're stressed out, we point to the people and events around us. When we have a "bad day," we cite a mean boss, an ungrateful child, a cancelled flight, a lousy waitperson, a flat tire, or the dog that ate our homework. When we're late, we point to the traffic.

It's important—pivotal actually—to understand that this excuse and blame game directly feeds our illusion of victimhood. It's so much easier, in the moment, to make excuses—to shift blame onto someone or something else—and then to wait for solutions that come from someone or something else. Aside from what this can do to our relationships with other people, this creates a dishonest relationship with ourselves and leads to a quiet, insidious undermining of our personal power. This is nothing less than tragic, because our personal power—our ability to live as empowered beings—is pivotal to our health and joy.

No one can wreck our day, or make us unhappy, or make our life hard. Don't get me wrong, I'm not suggesting you beat yourself up about your life experience, either—that's blame too, simply targeted at ourselves instead of something outside of us. But largely, other people are just being. Not always honestly, not always kindly, and not always collaboratively. But the only bus that I have control over is my own bus. I can't *make* my kid respect me, or *make* the cashier be pleasant, or *make* my boss appreciate me. By giving my power away to others, I'm simply telling myself that I'm powerless, a hapless victim. When we paint ourselves as the victim, it's our personal power that we're giving away. This has personal and global ramifications, none of them helpful or happy. This myth is so important that all of Chapter 3 is dedicated to helping you be large-and-in-charge in your life experience.

Myth: Money Fixes Everything

The Europeans who sailed across the pond to populate America were people driven to create abundance, pursue freedom, and build good lives for themselves. (They were also driven in a way that left little room for regard or respect of the people and animals that were already here.) Generations later, we're still driven by those same impulses, even though we're well beyond the success, ease, and self-reliance those early Americans came to create. We continue to blindly pursue more success and wealth without defining what, exactly, those words mean to us. And it's making us miserable.

Like most of us, I used to think that when I had more money, things would be better. I'd have less stress, more time, better health, and be happier. Instead, I've discovered that what we want isn't money: it's the power to do what we want with our lives. We want the power of choice. Because money can often afford power and choice, we think that by getting money, we'll be happy. We think that money fixes everything. But this popular myth is similar to the weight myth. Meaning, many of us believe that we'll be happy, and feel good about ourselves, when we lose weight. Yet when we lose the weight, our insecurities and self-worth remain unchanged, so we're simply a slimmer version of our unhappy selves. Similarly, when we attain wealth, we'll still be the same person inside that we are today, with the same values, tools, and mindset. We'll simply be a more financially wealthy person with the identical internal issues that we started out with. Money can certainly help, but it doesn't fix everything.

Myth: Addiction Is a Niche Issue

Our modern-day struggle with addiction is another one of those common-but-not-normal myths that we've become blind to as a society. And it's a deeply personal issue for people. When we hear the word *addiction*, we tend to think about people starting their day with a twelve-pack, heroin overdoses, or someone blowing their family savings at a casino. Alcohol, heroin, and gambling are indeed famously and ruinously addictive; however, almost anything can become addictive. The most common addictions are work, sex, food, consumerism (shopping), gambling, internet, social media, power, personal looks (including plastic surgery addiction), caffeine, nicotine, alcohol, and other drugs (illegal and prescribed).

However, focusing on the forms through which addiction expresses itself is, in many ways, a misguided discussion. The question is what is the source—the genesis—of these self-destructive addictive behaviors? Most science and schools of psychology point to **trauma**. Addiction is the behavior, and trauma is the root cause of behavior. We'll further explore trauma in Chapter 7, and trauma is a deeply misunderstood area of mind and mental health. Peter Levine, a clinical psychologist who specializes in trauma, said that "trauma is the most avoided, ignored, denied, misunderstood and untreated cause of human suffering." This leads to many unfortunate outcomes.

Various addictions garner societal acceptance or rejection along a continuum. It's become cool to be a work addict—folks half-joke about it in casual conversation—but if you're a single mom with three kids and a heroin addiction, then people purse their lips and shake their heads and wonder why you can't get your act together and be a good parent for chrissakes. In most of America, if you're addicted to material expression of wealth, you're looked up to as a rock star and people want to *be* you. They don't see the child inside who was abused at home, bullied at school, or was smaller than the other kids. They don't see that your only moments of fleeting happiness are when people are envying what you have. We don't see the pain behind the accepted addictions, and we judge the unaccepted addictions—although all of them are the same cry for help, packaged in a different form.

We have addictions because there is a wounded part of us that's hurting. On a deep level we don't feel equipped to deal with the pain of our trauma, so we're addicted to something (or several things) that numbs this pain. We rely on our addiction(s)-of-choice to deliver dopamine to our brain, creating a moment when we feel okay and in control. The rest of the time, when we're not engaged with our addiction, we don't feel good. We feel bad, or sad, or anxious, or empty, or broken, or worthless, or afraid, or most often some uncomfortable mixture of those feelings.

The root problem is that people are wounded, ashamed, and lonely. Via dopamine, they become wired to perpetuate the cycle of pain, most often in an increasingly addictive trajectory, as the addiction quickly becomes chemical as well as psychological. People struggling with addiction don't need our shaming and disdain; they need our compassion. We're making the people the problem, when in reality, it's something much bigger than the individual people: a cultural system that feeds addiction and then shames the addicted, while ignoring the invisible, unhealed wounds of trauma. Only the behavior is visible, and we inadvertently ignore the deeper wounds that elicit the behavior. This is a perfect segue into our final myth.

Myth: Solution-Based Solutions Are the Answer

The war on drugs, healthcare reform, addiction treatment, the war on cancer, diets for our ballooning obesity problem, and alleged reform via the prison system—these are some of the unsuccessful solutions to our widespread problems. Many of the solutions that we create are what I call *solution-based solutions*. They're related to the fact that we love the thrill of creating and marketing a solution, as opposed to loving the deep and complex work of foundationally solving problems. Solution-based solutions are akin to swatting at ants running around on our counter, even as we notice that their numbers seem to be increasing from some unseen source. We see ants, and we swat at ants. In contrast, a *problem-based solution* would be to roll up our sleeves and dig under the counter to learn garbage remnants and wood rot created an ant paradise. We see ants, and we seek to find the core contributing issue(s) to the exploding ant population in our kitchen. The solution-based solution of swatting at the ants is ineffective and is a lesson in frustration, yet this is often the kind of solution—big, expensive solutions—that we come up with.

Take the prison system. Putting people in a soul-sucking, dog-eat-dog prison and feeding them nutrient-deplete food comes from having a solution that derives from how we want things to end up—a solution-based solution. We want the "bad people" off the streets and separated into their own culture, where they can feel punished, which will cause them to mend their ways. As we've seen for decades, this doesn't work. Within a five-year period following incarceration, the re-arrest rate is around 77 percent, depending on the statistics source.

Don't get me wrong; it's good to know the goal for our solution, but it's important to include the uncomfortable harshness of reality: what are the actual problems? We can then base our solutions on the problems. Einstein once said that we can't solve a problem from the same kind of thinking that caused it, and he's right. People don't commit crimes because they need to be punished. Most people commit crimes because of trauma, mental illness, poverty, isolation, and, as it turns out, malnourishment. Although I certainly don't have the neatly packaged problem-based solution to reforming those who engage in criminal activity, I do know of one woman who did an interesting prison probation experiment that highlights what problem-based solutions can do.

Barbara Stitt worked as a probation officer in Ohio. Her book, *Food and Behavior: A Natural Connection*, outlined her on-the-ground experiments in drastically reducing the re-arrest rates of her probationers. Her problem-based solution? She re-imagined the rehabilitation process to include assessment of the individual's health; and the introduction of a corrective, healthful diet as a mandate during probation. In comparison to a re-arrest rate norm of 77 percent, the 5,000-plus probationers who came through her office had *an 11 percent re-arrest rate.*

Prison inmates are served the cheapest food possible: industrially-processed, nutrient-deplete food with a long shelf life. This food sends us into the lizard part of our brain where survival and violent urges reside. Not such a good idea anywhere, but especially in prison. You see, we've evolved to use our frontal lobe for problem solving, judgment, sexual behavior, reasoning, self-control, and decision-making. Prison food sends the incarcerated away from using their frontal lobe. Hmm. Replenishing the body (and brain) with nutrients brings us back to using the frontal lobe of our brain, in favor of self-regulation and ethical decision-making. Barbara devised a problem-based solution to reduce re-arrest rates. Imagine if nutritious food and trauma therapy were both required for the incarcerated. Problem-based solutions require more creativity and heavy lifting, but they tend to work, and these types of solutions are exactly what we'll be discussing in the coming chapters.

So Now What?

So here we are. A world heavily populated with wounded, isolated people who feel this never-ending pressure to have, do, and achieve. This pressure to relentlessly drive forward distracts us from our underlying wounds until we completely lose sight of ourselves in our rear-view mirror. Thus, many of us who have relative abundance find ourselves in the condition of being efficient, responsible, and well-informed—and at the same time dissatisfied, restless, and unhappy. This makes sense, of course, given all the cultural factors we've discussed. There is a deep pain in the chest of our modern culture that is so common that it's largely undiscussed and unaddressed. As the wise Indian philosopher Jiddu Krishnamurti purportedly said, "It is no measure of health to be well adjusted to a profoundly sick society." A wild world. So now what?

First, my hope is that with the common-but-not-normal brought into your viewfinder, you'll notice them more. Your perception of the world you live in may feel a little bit different. Maybe some of what you're seeing isn't so appealing to you. You and I have no control over the culture that we live in, but we do have immense control over the choices we make and how we choose to live our lives. We have power over how we care for ourselves, how we think, how we act, and what we support with our time and money. When we watch a news show, we're supporting that show with our time, which boosts their ratings, thus communicating to them, *Stay on track. I love what you're doing.* When we buy organic apples, we're telling the marketplace that we prefer our apples without pesticides. Many people voting the same way—with their money, actions, and time—eventually create a shift in the culture.

Yet, how do we cultivate and unlock our potential for health and joy in this culture that's constantly telling us that we're not good enough, that we're alone in our struggles, that people are scary and mean, that we're hapless victims, and that healing comes from outside of ourselves? The answer is a bit of a paradox.

My intent in this chapter was twofold. First, to encourage you to let yourself off the hook. Many of the people I work with feel down on themselves because they can't seem to lose weight, get healthier, kick habits, feel more satisfied, or get along with people important to them. I often start by pointing out how our culture can derail us without us even realizing. I share that we swim along in this water we can't see, feeling lousy about ourselves; dissatisfied with our life experience; lonely in our messiness; and often blaming things, people, and situations outside of ourselves for all of that muck. The first step in creating better health and more joy in our lives is to let ourselves off the hook for the past. We stop beating ourselves up.

Here's the paradox part: my second intent in this chapter was for us to have an idea of what we're letting ourselves off the hook for, so that we can now move from off-the-hook for the past to *full ownership going forward*. When we become aware of the water we're swimming in—of all the mythology that instructs our daily life—the only true solution is to break out of the prison of victimhood, find and step into our power, and begin to unlock our powerful human potential that's been there all along. To take personal responsibility for our entire life experience—body, mind, and spirit. You might ask, "How do I start such a pivotal change?"

CHAPTER 2:

CREATING HEALTH AND JOY

"The key is changing our habits and, in particular, the habits of our mind."
—PEMA CHÖDRÖN, BUDDHIST TEACHER

"Ninety-seven percent of you won't use what you learn at this three-day training to create the very change that you traveled for thousands of miles, and paid thousands of dollars, to get."

This is what I heard, several years ago, when I was at a conference in California. The speaker shared this "3 percent rule" on day one. His statement was blunt; and based on my previous speaking and conference experiences, it was also accurate. Unlocking our potential for health and joy is not simply about learning, understanding, reading a book, or taking a class. Taking in new information, new ways of looking at things, and cultivating understanding are certainly important aspects of our personal evolution. It's true that knowledge can be power. It's also true that we must set intentions and follow them with action. However, the magic in any personal evolution is about rewiring habits and beliefs. Personal evolution is about changing our minds. If you can change your mind, you can transform your life experience.

Want to eat healthy? Change your mind.

Want to improve your relationships? Change your mind.

Want to dedicate yourself to a fitness routine that makes you strong and that you thoroughly enjoy? Yup, you got it—change your mind.

If you don't get your mind on board, nothing else you try—from exercise to stress management to vegetables—will stick.

We're wired for evolution—to learn and grow as beings. If we weren't, we'd stay as infants, crawling around on all fours and wearing diapers. How can we evolve in a way that brings us the most health and joy?

Change Your Mind, Change Your Experience

Starting a discussion about change is not to say that there's anything wrong with you exactly the way you are. We're all perfectly imperfect. You are enough as you are. Yet, as we just talked about, we're also wired for *personal evolution*, a term I prefer over the term *personal development*. We're changing and evolving, whether we think about it or not. Some of us embrace the idea of personal evolution and engage with it intentionally as a worthwhile and exciting journey. Some of us evolve simply as a natural outcome of living on this planet, experiencing people and circumstances that change and shape us. The latter tends to happen more slowly and haphazardly, and often with more suffering. This isn't bad, per se, it's simply nonconscious evolution— evolution without intention. This book is a guide for our intentional evolution toward a more healthy, joyful life experience.

Whether you're interested in intentional personal evolution on a tiny scale, on a grand scale, or somewhere in between isn't important. If you're interested in being the owner and creator of your life experience, you must understand what lies at the center of it. Both our life experience and our personal evolution have a singular catalyst that is the creator and the destroyer, the facilitator and the obstructer, the barrier or the bridge—the mind. Thus, the only way to change our experience in life is through intentional use of the mind. When we change our mind, we change our experience.

The Three Amigos

Change can be hard. Embracing the new and releasing the familiar is challenging, even if we intellectually understand that the old, familiar way isn't working for us anymore. If we smoke two packs a day and start experiencing asthma, we may understand that the asthma is connected to the smoking. We also understand that if we stop smoking our body will invariably heal and it's unlikely we'll continue to suffer from asthma. However, the vast majority of people keep smoking. Not because they're stupid, lazy, or uninformed, but because change is hard and their thinking and physiology have become addicted to the cigarettes. Since the human experience and change can be hard, it's helpful to have amigos—Spanish for friends—to help out.

Every one of us has access to what I call the **Three Amigos**: awareness, curiosity, and mindfulness. We were born with them, and we use them full-throttle as children. However, as we age, we become socialized into leaving them inert in a filing drawer of our mind. We can reactivate these natural states. These amigos are also choices that we can make, each moment of our days so that they eventually "re-become" our default approach and support us in health, joy, and personal evolution. They support us in living the most deep and broad expression of our awesomeness. Developing awareness, curiosity, and mindfulness can assist us in all aspects of our lives and are fundamental to our journey together in this book. The Three Amigos are part of the bedrock that supports our ability to move into the fullest expression of our human majesty. Let's get refamiliarized with these innate life approaches.

Awareness is difficult to describe with words and to grasp with our intellect. Awareness is a slight shift in the way that we move through the world, where we move from life on automatic to noticing the-not-usually-noticed. Our perception of our environment, of others, and of ourselves becomes softer and wider to include subtleties that we might otherwise mentally dismiss.

A baby or young toddler notices everything around them. They're soaking in their environment, including people, with a sense of wonder. They don't have any preconceived notions; they're simply acutely aware of many things that we no longer notice as adults. These young beings default toward awareness. It's how they're learning about the planet that they've just come into. As adults, we can relearn this state of being by moving more slowly and by utilizing the other two of the Three Amigos.

Curiosity is an approach—to learning, to people, to challenges, and to life—that opens the heart and mind. Curiosity is soft around the edges. You can learn about curiosity by observing a six-month-old baby as she approaches the unknown and not-yet-understood. Watch as she picks up something new and turns it around and around, soaking in information and processing it, inviting input from all her senses to guide her on what she doesn't yet understand. She is aware and intent, yet soft and open. The reason babies approach learning this way is because it's the best way to learn, and they haven't yet had curiosity socialized out of them by fear, doubt, and the idea of "knowing" the answer. The most important thing we can do when facing challenges, confusion, adversity, confrontation, and lack of understanding is to cultivate this moment-to-moment curiosity.

It's amazing what we can do with curiosity, even in the most incongruent emotional spaces. If we can sit in the middle of chaos and cultivate curiosity, something shifts. We start to feel as if something is working with us rather than against us. We feel more collaborative and less combative. Curiosity allows us to open to possibilities, understanding, and wisdom that might never have come to us otherwise.

Developing our curiosity muscle, in most any application, allows us to become adept at the art of inquiry. Curiosity and the art of inquiry are common themes in this book, and they're less about finding "the answer" and more about the fascinating things we'll uncover on this learning adventure.

Often, we tend to approach things that we don't understand with the attitude of wanting to know what's right and what's wrong. Life, and everything in it, is much more rich, complex, and juicy than this. With the exception of certain clear moral and ethical questions, right and wrong most often aren't the interesting parts of life, or valid ones. Sometimes, things are both right *and* wrong, depending on how we look at them. Getting comfortable with paradox is helpful as we cultivate curiosity. Remember that lack of evidence doesn't always point to the evidence of lack. Our complex and nuanced world invites us to remain curious, even if—especially if—we think we've found the answer. Imagine if we hadn't remained curious and left our knowledge at the-world-is-flat.

Curiosity, and its associated art of inquiry, opens us to a different way of looking at things when our beliefs don't neatly line up with what's in front of us or what we're being told. This doesn't necessarily mean we're looking to change our beliefs, but simply that we're willing to explore and learn new things. It means that instead of seeing limitation, we see opportunity; instead of good or bad, we see interesting nuances; instead of better or lesser, we find a middle way that is more rich, instructive, and inclusive. Curiosity helps us cultivate a more open heart and mind and is fed by our first amigo, awareness and our third amigo, mindfulness.

Mindfulness is open, active attention to the present moment, with an awareness that the present moment simply IS. It's a conscious, purposeful way of tuning in to what's happening right now, within us and around us, without judgment. It's our basic ability to be fully present, aware of where we are and what we're doing. When we're mindful, we're not overly reactive or overwhelmed by what's going on around us. Mindfulness allows us to recognize our options, to respond instead of react. It gives us the power to change our past conditioning. It allows us deeper vision, with respect and compassion for what we see. It supports us in noticing when our hearts open and close to the people, circumstances, and events around us. Mindfulness allows us to non-judgmentally notice right where we are. It paves the way for fully conscious living—for us to purposefully create our personal reality and our personal evolution.

Mindfulness feeds, and is fed by, awareness and curiosity. Together they are the Three Amigos. They're loving friends for one another, and loving friends for you on your life journey. They'll support you in living with joy and intention. The Three Amigos assist you in using your mind in a more focused, productive way, which is a key creator of health and joy.

The Myth of Willpower

Many of us believe that the reason we struggle to implement change— to evolve toward the fullness of our being—is that we lack **willpower** or self-control. We're led to believe if we can just have enough willpower, then we'd be on the way to our goals. In truth, willpower is misunderstood and our modern society has a misguided view of willpower for two main reasons. First, our culture supports a false expectation that willpower solves problems. It doesn't. Second, we live in a pop-a-pill, liposuction, three-week diet, seven-second video, sound-bite culture that encourages us to want what's new, quick, and easy—which I call the silver bullet syndrome. Thus, willpower *seems* to be a quick and easy answer to getting healthier and more joyful, like a silver bullet.

Let's explore why our reliance on willpower to create lasting change is misguided, using the trusty metaphor of a rocket-launch. When we launch a rocket to the moon, a proportionally huge amount of fuel and power is used in the very beginning of the trip. This energy gets the giant thing off the launching pad, free from gravity, and through Earth's relatively dense atmosphere into space. The vast majority of the effort is expended in the first 0.17 percent of the trip, which is less than 1 percent of the journey. In contrast to Earth's atmosphere, outer space is more of a vacuum and allows for the relatively effortless continuation of travel. Put another way, the first 430 miles of the trip is where most of the effort is required, while the remaining 238,900 miles are a relative breeze.

You might see where I'm headed with this metaphor. When we launch any change in our lives, the tool of willpower simply gets us off the launching pad. A proportionally huge amount of energy and focused intention are used in the very beginning of the change to create new habits and to free ourselves of our old habits and beliefs, which are the gravity that pulls us back to what we know. This is equivalent to that first 430 miles for the rocket.

Once we move through "blast off," we've created new habits, and the change we've created is our new neurological set point. This is thanks to neuroplasticity (our brain's ability to change and reorganize itself by creating new neural connections throughout our life) and to our complex and powerful mind. Once we're in "outer space" and practicing our new habits, they require a relatively small amount of energy and mental power to keep them intact as a lifestyle choice. This is equivalent to the remaining 238,900 miles of the rocket's trip to the moon.

Willpower can be helpful in momentary behavior intervention—in the very beginning and during the twenty-one to sixty-six days of consistent action that's required to create habit change—but it's an exhaustible and exhausting resource. It's exhaustible in that we have only so much of it, and then it's used up and we can't call on it for help, and it's exhausting because it uses copious amounts of mental energy. Mental energy is associated with our brain and our mind; it's worth taking a quick tour through the brain and mind to understand why willpower is not the seat of change or of personal evolution.

Meet Your Brain and Mind

It's important to understand that the brain and the mind are different, albeit related, aspects of our humanness.

The **brain** is a complex and powerful physical organ that lives in your skull. It's the most complex object known to humankind. The brain is the command center for our nervous system and body functions; it also interfaces with our mind. In contrast, the **mind** does not *live* anywhere, as it's nonphysical. The mind is the seat of our humanness; it includes the felt sense of self, thought, our experiences, memory, as well as faculties like intuition.

It bestows our ability to be aware of the world. There are aspects of mind that we can loosely associate with areas of the brain, as the brain can act as a receptor for mind activity.

As we understand it, we have a conscious mind and a nonconscious mind. The **conscious mind** is the part of our psyche that includes direct awareness. It is where we experience ourselves and the environment directly through sensory experiences such as sight, sound, taste, hearing, touch, and mental activity. The **nonconscious mind** is our storage center, our autopilot, and the seat of our habits and beliefs. It engages with all mental activity that is not in our awareness.

Going forward, you'll find that I sometimes use the phrases **mind-brain**, or **mind-brain system**, which are the phrases most accurate in the many topics of inquiry where people are unclear on what is associated with mind versus brain. I use the term *mind-brain* because often, it's difficult to separate mind function from brain function, as they're deeply interdependent. My intent in providing the *Spark Notes* on brain and mind here is to help you fully grasp the limitations of willpower, and the power of habits and beliefs.

Willpower comes from our conscious mind, which comprises about 5 percent of our mental activity. The other 95 percent of our mental activity comes from our nonconscious mind, which is where our habits and beliefs reside. True, lasting change is maintained with habits and beliefs. Further, willpower seems to be associated with the prefrontal cortex of our brain, which is a new part of our brain from an evolutionary perspective. This means that our ability to override our desire in the moment, via willpower, is relatively new brain circuitry. Meanwhile, the ancient part of our brain that contains the limbic system, where our reward system lives, is partially controlled by dopamine, our I-want-to-feel-good-now neurotransmitter. This part of our brain holds our original wiring, and we revert to it when we're *tired, stressed, nutrient-depleted*, and/or *sleep-deprived*. That ancient dopamine reward system is also what fuels and sustains addiction, and it's a powerful system indeed.

Houston, we have a problem. Do you see that your frustration with creating sustained positive change in your life isn't in any way related to laziness or ineptitude? The issue is that you've been trying to override your large and powerful nonconscious mind and the longstanding and powerful reward system in your brain, by using your easily exhaustible, conscious willpower. This tiny faculty of willpower comes from your brain's new-kid-on-the-block (the prefrontal cortex) and is associated with less than 5 percent of your mental power. Further, we often attempt to utilize willpower when we're tired and stressed out. Willpower is ineffective when we're in that state because it requires significant mental energy, for starters. Further, when we're tired and stressed out, we're also operating more from the part of our brain that favors our ancient reward system. Trying to create change using willpower is akin to trying to dig the Panama Canal with a plastic spoon. This results in fits-and-starts, exhaustion, feelings of hopelessness, and you're likely to abandon the plan instead of realizing your desired outcomes.

When it comes to our health and joy, the questions are not:

1. "What do I want?"

2. "Where is my willpower?"

The questions are:

1. "What am I passionate enough about that I'm willing to endure the most disagreeable parts of the work for?"

If you're not willing to keep at it when the novelty of "doing something new" wears off, you won't stay on track for long.

2. "WHY do I want it?"

If you're not crystal clear on your deep-down, brass-tacks WHY, your commitment will wane quickly.

Willpower can be a helpful tool for behavior control *in the moment*, but it's not how we create lasting change. We must be clear about why we want something, and we must understand that if a quick fix were an option, we would've realized our desires long ago. Once we've gotten real on those two questions, we employ our mighty nonconscious mind to get traction toward our deepest desires. This is where the power of habit comes in.

The Truth of Habits

What do Oprah Winfrey, the 14th Dalai Lama, Georgia O'Keeffe, Warren Buffet, and LeBron James have in common? Anyone who's excelled at anything—sports, business, acting, meditation, art, media, financial wealth, friendships, parenting, badminton—is a master of habits and beliefs, and these well-known cultural icons are no exception. The lasting change that we *can't* get from willpower, we *can* get from intentionally created habits and beliefs. As our brilliant Greek brother Aristotle wrote, "We are what we repeatedly do. Excellence, then, is not an act, but a habit." There are two kinds of habits: habits of action and habits of thought. These two types of habits affect each other, and they warrant some exploration.

What, exactly, is a **habit**? A habit is an action, routine, thought, or behavior that we perform regularly and often automatically. It's estimated that 40 to 50 percent of our actions are run by habits. That all sounds okay, right? It's nice to not have to think about every single thing we do. Can you imagine always tying your shoelaces the same way you did the first time you tried it? Habits save time and mental energy, so bravo for habits. But there's a hitch: without the exhaustive and exhausting intentional intervention of willpower, our brain defaults to the path of least resistance—habit. It's postulated that each day, we make more than 200 habitual choices just about eating. Habits control what we eat, yes, and almost every aspect of our lives as well. I'd wager that you don't get up in the morning and ponder whether to brush your teeth, or whether you'll get dressed or not. These are habits. Okay, the latter one is also sort of a legal issue since we can get arrested for public nudity in some parts of the world, but there are no laws about dental hygiene. We brush our teeth anyway because it's habit. This doesn't mean that we never, ever skip brushing our teeth or that we should chastise ourselves when we don't. It simply means that it's something that we typically do, without thinking much about it, which is a habit.

Driving a car is a process requiring a myriad of actions. When we first learn to drive, it seems difficult and tiring, with so many things to remember. Once we practice and create habits—such as turning on our directional signal any time we're going to make a turn, or taking our foot off the gas the second we see brake lights—it becomes easier. This is largely because driving becomes a collection of habits that is run by our nonconscious mind. Further, when we drive a route over and over, we don't even need to think about how to get there. Have you ever come to the end of a drive and realized that you don't remember *a single thing* about your drive? While driving, your mind was preoccupied with thinking or with focusing on your music, and you made hundreds of decisions using your autopiloted habits. Truly amazing. Habits are powerful; they become hardwired into our mind and our neurocircuitry, so that we don't have to actively think about them. Habits are our mind-brain system's way of increasing efficiency, which is great. What's not so great are the parts of that programming that work against us, such as reaching for sweets or crunchy, empty carbs whenever we've had a challenging day.

Beliefs are habits of thought. They are thoughts that we think over and over again until they become our personal belief system. Many of the beliefs we hold stem from programming that we received from other people. In fact, the bulk of our core beliefs were programmed *for us* by the time we turned seven, and these were other people's programs that were either forced upon us or that we soaked up like little human sponges. Even when we're intentionally avoiding those early programmed beliefs, input such as colors, tastes, sounds, music, circumstances, and feelings can all trigger ancient programs to take over again. Hence, at a basic level, the way in which we view life, and the way in which we interact with others, is based on other people's programs that got downloaded into our hard drive. This can turn out to be a real bummer.

For instance, someone who grows up with a reactive, angry parent may end up with the programmed belief that, *"I am someone who makes people angry. There is something very wrong with me, that I somehow provoke such angry outrages in people."* When in fact, the parent's reactivity and anger had everything to do with their own belief systems that might have been wired largely in their own childhood, and has nothing to do with their child. But what we believe about ourselves in childhood often becomes our personal dogma, and it can go either way. Meaning, in contrast to the person who grows up with a reactive, angry parent, if someone's childhood is rich in feedback that they can achieve whatever they set out to do, they can grow up with that positive belief. Even if their intellect, or conscious mind, runs into many examples that conflict with that idea, their belief of positive self-worth will stay strong. It's nonconscious programming that runs the show. Some of our beliefs are healthy and supportive, opening our heart and encouraging positive self-worth:

"I'm worth my own effort."

"I can be or do anything."

"People are wired for love and connection."

"I'm doing my best, and my best is good enough."

"My food choices matter."

"My body is beautiful and self-healing."

"I can, and will, make a difference."

Some of our beliefs narrow our perspective, close our hearts, and erode our self-worth:

"I'm not worth my own effort, or anyone else's."

"I'm not good/smart/savvy enough to do _____."

"People are selfish and cruel."

"Money is bad."

"Money will make me happy."

"Only skinny people can be happy."

"I can't possibly make a difference."

These are all beliefs. Know this: a thought that passes through our mind is harmless unless we believe in it. It's not our thoughts, but the attachment to our thoughts, our believing them without inquiry, and our judgment that cause suffering. A thought can be simple: *My buddy didn't return my phone call*. And then if we add on creative stories that ripple from our belief systems like: *My buddy didn't return my phone call because he's wrapped up in his new friends at work and he probably thinks he's too cool for me now* we'll start to accept these "proofs" of our beliefs without questioning. We're often invested in the belief that we're the authority on How Life Is, and our views become calcified around our old and often inaccurate beliefs—even though we aren't the author of most of them. Most of our concepts and philosophies are based on a lifetime of uninvestigated beliefs.

Not understanding all of this is exactly how we stay stuck and unable to change, and then, even more damaging than the actual stuck-ness, we feel bad about ourselves because of the stuck-ness. We did the diet and fell off the wagon. We didn't yell at our challenging child for a whole day, and then we blew our top. We started a meditation practice and, after a few frustrating days of trying, we stopped. Shifting habits and beliefs is a big part of my work with people, and it's an expansive subject. Here's what's most important: you need to understand that our nonconscious mind is powerful, and it operates largely outside of our conscious radar.

While we can't outrun our nonconscious mind any more than we can outrun our shadow, we can reprogram it. We can change our habits, of action and mind, to align with our desires for health, joy, and personal evolution. In 1949, neuropsychologist Dr. Donald Hebb postulated that "neurons that fire together, wire together," which eventually became known as Hebb's Law. A neuron is a specialized cell that transmits various types of information and communication within the body at up to 390 feet per second between itself and the other 86-plus billion neurons in our body (including our brain). Hebb's Law says that through repeated intervention in our actions and thoughts, we can rewire our mind-brain. Even though some research shows that our old habits don't disappear completely, they can become overpowered by our new, intentional habits. These new habits can take anywhere from twenty-one to sixty-six days to root in our mind-brain system. A key fulcrum of harnessing the power of our mind lies in mastering these nonconscious habits of thought and action, and learning to tend them as a gardener who weeds out some plants, while encouraging others—frequently and with love.

Rewiring 101

How do we do that? How do we create new habits? These are splendid questions because our mind is the bridge or the barrier to all that we want from life, the vast majority of which can be categorized under health, joy, or personal evolution. Our habits (of action) and our beliefs (habits of thought) are a key part of this bridge-barrier aspect of mind.

Before we get into the rewiring discussion, there are two important nuances of habits that you must understand. One nuance is "effective or ineffective habits"; the second (related) nuance is "people labels."

I'm not a fan of pulling in subjective judgment to label habits as either good habits or bad habits, as the phrase "bad habit" often triggers unnecessary shame. More accurate, and less damning, is the idea of "effective habits" and "ineffective habits." Is this habit effective or ineffective *in helping me create my best life experience?* This means that the habit needs to be looked at from a holistic perspective. For instance, let's say I have a habit of sitting on the couch and turning on Netflix during the time of day when I also have the opportunity to go for a run. Let's also say that improving my cardiovascular health is a top goal of mine. Therefore, it's not that Netflix is necessarily a bad habit; it's instead an ineffective habit, at that time of the day, for my goals. However, if my goal was to start my own streaming service, then spending time checking out what market leaders like Netflix are doing would be an effective habit. Hence, the effectiveness or ineffectiveness of my habits is contextual to my desired outcomes and the time of the day.

Similarly, habits aren't accurate labels of people. Habits don't define who we are. Smoking cigarettes doesn't denote moral weakness; it denotes a routine that follows a cue, which has led to psychological and chemical addiction. There's nothing moral or immoral about it. It's wiring. I chose cigarettes as an example because they're notoriously addictive and unhealthy. Notice I didn't say that they're ineffective for everyone. If someone doesn't care at all about their health and cares a lot about relaxation, and smoking brings them the reward of relaxation, then it's an effective habit. However, it's a rare person who would choose to die from lung cancer, or to live with emphysema and pulmonary disorder. It's important to be honest with ourselves about our goals.

Let's explore the key steps of the rewiring process, so that you can use them as you work with the concepts and ideas in the remaining chapters. With habits, there are generally two situations we find ourselves in. One is that we simply want to create a new habit. For instance, maybe we've learned that meditation is an effective promoter of whole-person health, and we want to incorporate it into our life. This situation asks that we create new circuitry and habits in our mind-brain to support a meditation practice. The second situation is that we have a current habit that is ineffective in supporting our intentions, and we want to override it with an effective habit. With either of these situations, our goal is to create a new habit that is effective in supporting our well-being.

Remember, this habit discussion is a major ingredient of the secret sauce that you'll use to create the health and joy you desire. To bring this information home and outline clear steps for habit creation, let's look at a real-life example from my client work.

Cora came to me because she wanted to lose weight. She was a fifty-something married mother of three teenage boys who was a partner in a law firm. Despite her repeated attempts to lose weight, she was now sixty pounds overweight and felt trapped in a body she didn't recognize, relate to, or feel good in. She also was experiencing symptoms related to being overweight such as frequent headaches, fatigue, and digestive discomfort. Given all that she'd achieved in her life, she couldn't understand why this important health change eluded her. She had reached the point of feeling hopeless when a longtime college friend told her about my work. To Cora's surprise, the first thing I honed in on during her intake process wasn't her health history, her lab results, or her food diary—it was her evening routines.

Cora's job entails a fair amount of stressors, and after a long day at work and then dinner with her family, she would sit in her home office and go through emails—and munch on crunchy, empty-carb snacks. This evening set of habits prolonged her work stress, contributed extra calories with no nutritive value to her body, and allowed no time for self-care and relaxation. Chronic stress creates a continual flow of fight-or-flight hormones in our body, and these hormones, if activated on a continual basis, lead to weight gain. Eating food for entertainment, especially after finishing a meal, adds unnecessary caloric intake. Lack of self-care and relaxation inhibits our feelings of well-being, which act to cement limiting thoughts we have about ourselves and our ability to lose weight. Each of these three outcomes was in direct opposition to Cora's goal to lose weight; so her post-dinner email time was not an effective habit for her goals.

STEP 1: EXAMINE

The first step with Cora was to lean in with curiosity and examine the existing situation:

Me: "What are you looking to achieve with your current evening habit?"

Cora: "I want to feel productive and to relax after dinner."

Me: "What change in your life experience do you want to create?"

Cora: "I want to lose weight and feel better."

Me: "Is the current habit effective in helping you create the change you want in your life experience?"

Cora: "No."

In the 1990s, researchers from the Massachusetts Institute of Technology uncovered a neurological process at the core of every habit, a three-step feedback loop that is hard-wired into our mind-brain. It's important to learn about and honor this process when understanding our habits so we can then create habit change. The three-step loop is:

Cue: any trigger that tells our brain which habit to use and when to use it.

A cue creates craving, which is marked by an increase of the neurotransmitter dopamine. Dopamine (and other neurotransmitters) is released when we anticipate *or* experience pleasure, and it demands reward.

Routine: is an activity, emotion, or behavior.

Reward: how our brain decides if the feedback loop feels beneficial to us or not.

The cue and the reward are powerful bookends and are key to figuring out next steps to changing the routine. Cues can be slippery buggers, so spend some time in figuring out what compels your activity, emotion, or behavior. Carefully observe your behavior over time and take notes. What were you doing when the ineffective habit kicked in? What were you feeling? What reward were you after?

Threading back to Cora's story, we use the questions that we asked in examining the current situation to help us suss out cue, routine, and reward.

Cue: Cora is seeking pleasure and productivity after dinner.

Routine: She grabs a bag of crunchy snacks and her laptop and settles into her home office.

Reward: She feels productive *and* like she's relaxing (when in reality she's not fully doing either).

It's amazing what dispassionate clarity comes from unpacking habits this way. In order to find an effective habit, the cue and the reward need to remain the same, or the brain will think the loop isn't working anymore. In Cora's case this would simply reinforce her desire for bags of crunch and a few more hours of perceived productivity on her laptop. *Changing the routine is where the magic lies.*

With this information, Cora and I worked to devise a new routine that would replace the ineffective after-dinner habit with an effective one. The new routine needed to fully support her goals for weight loss as well as give her the reward of feeling productive and relaxed after dinner. Her cue remained the same: finishing dinner. So, her new routine following her meal was to allow her husband to clean up while she made a mug of her favorite herbal tea. In addition, she began to put ten dark-chocolate-covered almonds in a pretty dish and get her laptop. Then, Cora and her husband would settle on the couch, setting a timer for twenty minutes. During that time, Cora drank her tea and got her delightful crunch on. She also got to go through email, flagging those to attend to first thing at the office tomorrow and briefly answering any that were urgent. Once the timer went off, she had to close the laptop and enjoy her tea and nutritious, metabolism-boosting crunch, while she and her husband watched TV, talked about their day, or played chess together.

STEP 2: ENVIRONMENT

The **environment** in which organisms and events unfold is foundational to results. Whether we're raising a child, growing a garden, healing disease, or studying what turns aspects of our genetics on and off—environment is everything. This truth is woven throughout the fabric of our lives. It's difficult to create change without assessing environment. In the context of habits, trying to create a new routine without making some change to the environment in which the old routine happens is setting yourself up for failure. How can you change your environment to support your goals and your new routine?

Changing physical location for a new routine can help make the change easier. Prepping our environment to support our goals is key, and small changes can make a big difference. These changes in our environment, and our relationship to our environment, set us up for success. Cora's environment needed to change in a few ways. She needed to remove the bagged snacks from her kitchen, making them unavailable at night, while being sure to stock her beloved chocolate-covered almonds and teas. Her routine needed to move to a new location of the house, and she needed to incorporate a timer to support her in limiting her work time. Finally, her environment needed to include activities other than work that helped her achieve her reward of feeling productive and relaxed.

Remember: environment is everything. As a parent, a cell biologist, and a gardener, I've come to understand that a child's behavior, a cell's integrity, or a plant's health all depend on their environment. Fix the environment of an organism, or the environment in which events take place, and form will follow function. In creating effective habits, we want our environment to make effective habits easy and ineffective habits hard.

STEP 3: REPROGRAM

There are many aspects to reprogramming habits, the most important of which is consistency. Earlier I mentioned that it takes twenty-one to sixty-six days to create a new, intentional habit. But habits form based on frequency, not time. If over sixty-six days, I do my new routine once or even fifteen times, I won't likely create a habit. If, however, I commit to getting my environment in order to support my new routine and do it every single day for sixty days, then I will likely succeed.

Part of consistency is making sure you don't interrupt your new routine. If that happens and you find yourself back in your old routine one day, I suggest the guideline of only one "miss." If you fall out of your habit on Wednesday, get right back in the saddle on Thursday.

For instance, my past attempts to create a meditation practice hadn't been successful, and I noticed that I often allowed many missed days to string together. I finally made meditation part of my health and joy practices when I got serious about my routine and accompanying environment. I created an effective environment by sitting in the same spot to meditate, using a guided meditation that was twenty minutes, every day for forty-five days. I only missed three nonconsecutive days during that time. Each day after meditation, I would mark an "M" on the small calendar that I keep in my purse. This type of habit tracking is effective and helps us keep it real with ourselves about how closely we're sticking to our new routine.

Keeping consistency with our routines to build effective habits is important because effective and ineffective habits are self-promoting. When we stick to our intentions for creating a new habit, we feel good about ourselves; this further amplifies our desire to stick to our habit-building intentions. Unfortunately, the reverse is also true. When we fall off the wagon and string several incidences together when we lean into our old routine, we feel badly about ourselves, which can lead us to lean more into our old routines for comfort. That said, if we do find ourselves off track for several days, we need to be kind with ourselves, and then simply hop right back into our new routine

CREATING HEALTH AND JOY | *51*

with a little boost from willpower. Neuroscience has shown that when we stray from our intentions and then berate ourselves for it, we're actually more likely to repeat the ineffective habit again. This thwarts our habit creation, and therefore our desire to move toward health and joy. We'll also miss out on all of that compound interest.

Small Things Are Big Things

Better health, a more calm and focused mind, weight loss, less drama, more joy and meaning, better relationships, and more—these results are the compound interest we gain from intentional investment in our habits. Compound interest is a financial term that refers to a little of something turning into a lot of something. If someone starts investing fifteen dollars a day at age twenty-five, they'll be a millionaire at a retirement age of around sixty-five, depending on their investment portfolio. Similarly, investing your time and energy in small habit changes can yield big results. These small habit changes seem more doable to our notoriously resistant mind, which is quite happy with the old, familiar, ineffective habit, thank you very much. Every tiny habit not only compounds to create palpable shifts in your personal evolution, but they also teach you one of the most important lessons: to trust yourself. Each of our habits and actions is a vote that we take about how we want to live, create, and relate to others in this lifetime. Another client of mine helped me see how life-altering a tiny habit change can be.

Dan came to me on orders from his wife, who was alarmed at his slide into obesity and poor health. He was unhappy to be meeting with me. Not the best-case scenario for helping someone. I met this challenge by creating a win/win/win. I asked Dan, "How about if I give you one, and only one, small new habit to adopt, that will improve many aspects of your health? Your wife will be happy that you're taking steps, you'll be happy that it's only one small change to make, and I'll be happy because I know this will make a significant difference for your physical health." Dan was hesitant but agreed. The one change that Dan made was to swap out his twelve ounces of morning orange juice for water; in ten months, he lost seventeen pounds and his diabetes markers improved. He was pretty excited. He was still doing many, many things that didn't support his well-being, but this one small consistent change added up to big results. Dan created a small new habit—what I call a micromovement—to move toward better health and more joy.

The Magic of Micromovements

Micromovements are tiny habits—actions and thoughts—that we consistently repeat to move toward our goals and desires. If you want to get to work on time each day, you start with an assessment of how much time it takes you to get physically ready to leave the house and then how long it realistically will take you to get to your office. Your first micromovement would be to set your alarm, every night, to accommodate that schedule. Your next micromovement might be to do any ironing the night before, and so on. These small actions work together to support bigger changes.

It doesn't work to say, *"Okay self, from now on, I'm going to _____."* Whether you're wanting to get to work on time, eat more health-building foods, exercise, or spend more time with your kids, you haven't made a plan. You're simply stating your desire. We need to craft and follow a series of sustained micromovements—new routines—to achieve our goals. These actions lead to new programming in our nonconscious mind that will do our heavy lifting for us, without effort or willpower, every day. Further, the bonus prize with micromovements is that, as we stick with each tiny step, we end up empowering ourselves with our actions. Day after day, our micromovements move us toward our desires, while building lasting habits and proving to ourselves that we can do it.

I know that it may not sound cool that a powerful, heart-centered woman like Oprah or a superstar athlete such as LeBron has micromovements, habits, and beliefs at the root of their success, but trust me, it's cooler than it seems at first blush. These folks work hard at what they consciously want to manifest, putting rock-solid habits in place that employ their powerful nonconscious mind. This amount of effort seems less cool than, *"I went to hear a motivational speaker last night and I feel superhuman today."* But what happens when real life steps in and that superhuman feeling that stoked our willpower is gone by lunchtime? Answer: nothing happens. That person is no closer to living their potential of the most healthy, joyful version of themselves that they can be. Willpower and motivation have their place. They are perfect for ignition and for intermittent behavior control. We just can't rely on them to create lasting change in our lives.

The real secret sauce for change lies in our habits. We must have a clear passion for the change; have a laser-accurate understanding of why we want the change; create new routines that satisfy the cue and reward feedback loop; tend a supportive environment; and then micromovement our way toward our desires.

The powerful thing about micromovements is that each little positive change invites more positive change, in a slow and steady movement toward what we desire. The challenging part is that our silver-bullet culture convinces us that change is easy, and it's not. However, the inconvenient truth is that if you are somewhere on a continuum of feeling lousy, dissatisfied, wounded, overweight, unhealthy, tired, and/or vaguely discontent, then change is the only way to get *out* of that. More of the same is simply going to create more of the same. The great news is that micromovements can create huge changes over time.

Unlock Your Potential

Now is where the rubber meets the road on our exquisite exploration. You understand more about the inner workings of our culture that work against you. You've explored the power of mind and how creating effective habits generates compound interest and moves you toward health and joy. Now we'll put all of that to good use.

If we want to live in a healthy body, we must take full responsibility for it, and reclaim our self-worth while nourishing our body and mind with self-care. We need to have some understanding of how the body works, how the body moves into dis-ease, and then how we can build health. We're best served by learning to use our complex and powerful mind as a tool—as a bridge to what we desire—instead of being slave to stress, drama, and emotional roller coasters. The strength of our connection to our spirit—the part of us that inhabits, and then eventually leaves, our body—has yet another level of effect on our health and state of joy and contentment.

How do we accept ourselves as we are, while also moving into an ever more full expression of our potential? The genesis of change lies in our mind. Habits, beliefs, and micromovements are the tugboats that ferry us toward our most magnificent selves.

The best place to start the next leg of our journey together to you unlocking your potential is with the foundational and vital pillars that will support you.

PART ONE

THE PILLARS: VITAL FOUNDATIONS

This section of the book is about love—self-love. Investing our time and attention to create empowered well-being isn't selfish, it's essential. This is akin to using an oxygen mask in-flight, where attending to yourself is not only beneficial to you but ends up benefitting those around you as well. It's all about the Three Pillars that we can build and strengthen in order to experience a more healthy and joyful life: *personal responsibility, self-worth,* and *self-care.*

These pillars are the vital foundations of being a balanced, healthy, whole person who's empowered to mindfully engage with life and its inherent joys, disappointments, passions, sorrows, fun, growth, responsibilities, pain, and relationships.

Most often when we talk about foundations they're cast as boring stuff that we have to suffer through to get to the cool desires that we really want. Before we can move through our life and exercise and play sports and hike mountains and participate in all kinds of fun and rewarding activities, we have to learn to walk. Before we build a house with its brilliant floor plan, details, paint colors, and functionality—and maybe even a Jacuzzi bathtub and a pool table—we have to build a solid foundation on which to create all those things. Before we can read and write and go to school and research and write love letters and take the bar exam, we have to learn the alphabet. Examples abound of how foundations get the bad rap of being humdrum, boring, mundane—a means to an end that we then forget about once we get our heart's desire (a spot on the soccer team, a steady income, or a better relationship). But all of that cool stuff can't happen without a solid foundation.

I'm here to tell you that foundations are a vital part of most everything we engage with. The trick is to approach foundational learning or foundational change with attention, dedication, and reverence—like you can't move on without it (because you actually can't). Know too that once you move on to the "cool stuff," you must keep tending that foundation to ensure it stays functional, solid, and supportive.

For example, in my work—that is, helping folks unlock their potential for health, joy, and personal evolution—food is often one of the first topics I discuss with my clients. Food is a powerful vehicle for change, and our physical and mental health often respond quickly to shifts that we make toward more nutrient-dense foods. Food is foundational to supporting our BodyMindSpirit, and we'll discuss it in more detail in Chapter 6.

Many years back, I was giving a four-week online class on food basics. A student named Kathy, along with her husband, took one piece of vital information about sugar intake from that class and ran with it. Months later, she wrote me to say that she and her husband had both lost weight, were sleeping better, and had more energy; she also experienced relief from the brain fog that had been dragging her down. She was amazed at this, given that they'd only changed that one thing.

In class, I'd explained what sugar does in the body; how it affects the mind-brain, including its addictive quality; and how to read the nutrition facts on the labels of packaged food. Kathy and her husband had read labels previously but had no frame of reference for the information. They now understood that four grams of sugar equals a teaspoon of sugar, and teaspoons are easier for us to relate to than grams. I had also explained that, for optimal health, the daily adult upper limit for sugar intake is about thirty-two grams, or eight teaspoons. Kathy and her husband had a few long food-shopping trips, reading labels and making changes to support their new foundational food tenet. After that, these new choices simply became habit. This simple change helped them make significant positive changes to their health picture, and to their understanding that foundations are vital and powerful. First up for vital foundations? Personal responsibility, a real game-changer.

CHAPTER 3:

THE PERSONAL RESPONSIBILITY PILLAR: OWN IT

"In the long run, we shape our lives, and we shape ourselves. The process never ends until we die. And the choices we make are ultimately our own responsibility."

—ELEANOR ROOSEVELT

"If you could kick the person in the pants responsible for most of your trouble, you wouldn't sit for a month."

—THEODORE ROOSEVELT

I spent a fair chunk of my life blaming personal challenges on my dad. It was his fault that I had low self-worth; that I was a perfectionist; that I craved validation from men; and that when people got irrationally angry with me, I shut down. This attitude of victimhood and blame infiltrated my life and had far-reaching effects in small and big ways. Further, while I was busy doing all that blaming, I was blind to the great things I had learned from my dad.

I've come to understand that most of us have felt this way at one time or another—that someone or something was keeping us from a happy existence. Maybe, like me, you've blamed someone or something else for your unhappiness or your bad behavior. Maybe you blame your genetics for your health problems. Maybe your blame your boss or co-workers for your lack of career advancement. Our list of blame stories is long and varied, and the singular, often-missed common denominator in all these stories is *ourselves.*

Chapter 1's section on the myth of the hapless victim explored how our freedom to be our most awesome selves is severely hobbled by labeling ourselves—mentally, conversationally, emotionally—as a victim. It's debilitating to label ourselves victims to life and to the people and experiences outside of ourselves. I'm here to tell you that there's only one creator of your life experience: you. Fully owning this creator role will unlock the doors to your health, joy, and personal evolution. This is why personal responsibility is the first pillar to engage, as it's the key to all that follows in this book, and in our lives.

Responsibility means being accountable for what we think, say, and do. If we play around with the word *responsibility,* we can pull out the two words: *response* and *ability*, which point to our *ability* to *respond* to our environment through conscious choice, since we possess the ability to pause, reflect, and choose our response. Our personal response-ability is an underused tool and an effective pillar that can be the fulcrum our whole life experience starts to turn and improve on. While this is true, there's a required mindset shift that must happen first which can be challenging for people, and it's this: we're personally responsible for our experience of everything that happens in our life. Have you ever been caught off guard by another's words or actions, responded defensively, and felt pissed off for the rest of the day about how they wronged you? Or complained for years about a job that you continued to stay in? What about feeling that your _____ (mother, ex-spouse, father, thankless child, etc.) is the root of most of your woes?

You're not alone in imagining that life is hard due to circumstances beyond your control. Here are four steps that have the power to lift us out of that hapless victim quagmire:

Step 1. Acknowledge: Play the No-Blame Game

As hard as it can be, instead of citing blame and excuses, we must *ACKNOWLEDGE*. If there is any part of our life experience we're not happy with, we acknowledge that we could make it different. Sometime this means acknowledging that we could work harder to get communication right, or we could work on being less selfish and mean, that we could take steps to be part of the solution rather than the problem, or that we could invest a little more in our well-being. The key is to acknowledge these things without making excuses. We must acknowledge our ignorance, lack of awareness, laziness, fear, or risk aversion. We acknowledge that apathy and failing sometimes seem better, on some level, than trying and failing. When blame and excuses and guilt come up, we must know that these are self-defeating "tools" we've developed to avoid the difficulties, embarrassment, or shame that can be involved with tackling the reasons, the real issues.

It's important to note that acknowledging is simply that: acknowledgment and moving on. This is NOT a directive to acknowledge and feel guilty, self-flagellate, or self-hate. Acknowledge does not mean that we blame ourselves. Self-blaming helps nothing; blame is part of the victim mentality. If you blame yourself, you become a victim of yourself and your imperfections; this does nothing to improve either your mood or your life situation. Beating ourselves up makes things worse, making it more likely that we'll do that self-defeating thing again in the future. Let's look at how this played out for a particular client of mine:

Peggy, similar to many people, struggled with emotional eating. She found herself nearing her fortieth birthday saddled with sixty-five extra pounds and a newly minted type 2 diabetes diagnosis. We needed to start our work together by helping Peggy develop a new relationship with food. I don't believe in rigidity, and I work with people to create a realistic health-promoting food lifestyle that's sustainable. Peggy did well for several weeks and then, as is inevitable, she slipped on the proverbial banana peel. Instead of a banana, however, it was an entire sleeve of Oreos. During her next appointment after the Oreo fiasco, Peggy confessed, simply dripping with shame, what happened. (Honestly, we can be so unforgiving with ourselves.) I explained to Peggy that when she falls off the wagon—notice I say *when* she falls off, not *if* she falls off—the absolute worst thing she can do is to berate herself. I told her that neuroscience has shown that when we berate ourselves for our mistakes, we increase the chances that we'll do it again. We're programming failure. Every cell in our bodies is continually eavesdropping on our thoughts. That's right, all fifty trillion cells are continually receiving signals and data from the environment of our body and mind, and then acting on that info:

Peggy: "UGH. I can't believe I just ate that whole sleeve of Oreos. I don't know how that happened! And I was doing so well. I suck. I'm never going to lose this weight. I have no self-control."

Peggy's cells: "Geez. Did everybody in here hear that? We're part of a person who sucks and has no self-control. Everyone got that? Let's make it happen!"

Instead of this self-hate, we're best served by dispassionately acknowledging what went awry so that we can educate ourselves about what's getting in our way. Next, we move on to Focus.

Step 2. Focus: Identify Your Circle of Influence

Once you've *acknowledged* the reason that any part of your life experience is different from what you want, the next step is to FOCUS. This is where we parse out what, if anything, we can do about it.

You can't change anything outside of yourself. The weather, your boss's ineptitude, your child's addiction, your partner's laziness, the season, the traffic, the state of the world, the political climate—most circumstances are largely outside of your circle of influence. The late, great Stephen Covey, who was the author and creator of the widely popular *7 Habits* books and trainings, explored the ideas of our circle of influence and circle of concern in *The 7 Habits of Highly Effective People.*

Imagine a big circle and call it your **circle of concern**. Here lives the vast array of things that we want to change: the rot on our front door, global warming, our kid's social circle, our partner's snoring, the political climate, our finances, gas prices, our loud neighbor's grating voice, you name it. Now imagine a much smaller circle nested in the center of that bigger circle and call it your **circle of influence**. Here lives the tiny array of things that we can affect: our attitude, intentions, perception, money management, and the rot on our front door. The illusion that we can control anything outside of our circle of influence serves to keep us miserable and victimized. As we wake up from that illusion, we see that there are many, many more things that we're concerned about than things we can directly influence.

For example, I would prefer that my teenage sons would not get involved with addictive substances. This desire is a big one for me and has logged significant frequent flyer miles in my circle of concern, especially as the opioid crisis continues to escalate. The only way I can bring this desire into my circle of influence, in any way, is to maintain an open dialogue with my sons about drug use. End of story. They make their own choices every day, and the majority of their time is spent out and about—at school, at work, with their sports teams, or with friends—not under my wing. I can't make their decisions for them, nor should I. Recognizing this, and thinking about the circle of concern and the circle of influence, assists me in focusing my parenting energy constructively on creating an open dialogue, instead of destructively on worrying, hovering over my kids, and stressing. I feel empowered by focusing my energy in ways that feel constructive to me and recognizing that I'm not in control of anything except myself.

When we're not happy with a relationship, we might ask ourselves what we could do differently. When we're dissatisfied with our job, maybe we sit with some serious self-inquiry into what we like and what we don't like, and ferret out where we might have a conversation, or get some training, or look to swap responsibilities. When our family vacation is turning out to be lame, maybe we do what we can to remedy it while cultivating a change of attitude. Maybe we take a family survey, rearrange the schedule, and hit the reset button.

Every moment of each day, that reset button is available. Our attitude, our perception, and our mental approach are the three things that always lie within our circle of influence. This idea is humbling and empowering.

Step 3. Act: Unlock Your Potential as a Creator

Once we've *acknowledged* our 100 percent ownership of our life experience and become *focused* on what resides in our circle of influence, we're ready for mindful and effective ACTION. You are a powerful creator and with consistent mindful intention, you can create a life experience that you joyfully inhabit. We're best served when we make conscious choices from the mindset of a creator as opposed to that of a victim.

The **Victim Mindset** says, *"My life experience happens outside of me and 'at' me. My health and joy are created and directed by outside influences."* This mindset serves to dilute our mighty human potential, as we then continually look for answers outside of ourselves to liberate us from our discomfort, our dissatisfaction, and our pain. The **Creator Mindset** says, *"My life experience is built from the inside (of me) out. My mindset instructs my health, joy, and life experience."* The Creator Mindset expands our potential as we become empowered to create the life experience we desire. Let's check out some examples:

Victim Mindset: "There's nothing I can do about it."
Creator Mindset: "I'm going to explore all options and alternatives."

Victim Mindset: "Hey look, that's just the way I am; my parents screwed me up. Take it or leave it."
Creator Mindset: "I can choose a different approach. It will be really hard in the beginning, and I'd love your support."

Victim Mindset: "She ruined my whole day."
Creator Mindset: "Yes, she was rude, but I'm in charge of my own feelings and response."

The Creator Mindset is focused on personal mindset, versus outside perceived barriers, and uses the steps of:

Pause (to gain perspective) → Reflect (to consider choices) → Respond

For example, someone may slam the proverbial door in my face (and they have, and boy does it feel crappy). Focusing on them, their rejection of me, and how they "wrecked everything" puts me into a Victim Mindset. Instead of focusing on the closed door, I'm better served by shifting my perspective from looking for someone to blame into one of looking for an open window. This is how a man named Theodore Geisel could receive twenty-seven publisher rejections for his first book, *And to Think I Saw It on Mulberry Street*, and keep trying the various windows in the Mansion of Possibility until he found that twenty-eighth window (Vanguard Press). He pried that sucker open, wiggled in, and the rest is Dr. Seuss history. He was using the Creator Mindset. Like Dr. Seuss, don't let anyone else determine your ability and worth as a creator.

Step 4. Own It: Avoid Having a Big But

After we *acknowledge* our role in circumstances, *focus* on what we can influence, and take *action* with a Creator Mindset, we arrive at the scrumptious icing on the personal responsibility cake: OWNING IT.

Truth: lasting happiness, or what I prefer to call joy and contentment, doesn't come from any external event or source. The only way to create health, personal clarity, abundance, harmony, satisfaction, and joy in our life experience is to take 100 percent ownership of our life. We have to abandon excuses, our victim stories, and our blaming of other people and circumstances—all the alleged reasons why our life experience is not what we want. Putting these behind us is the only way to create change, achieve success, cultivate happiness, and to love our life. We have the ultimate power to direct our mindset, and ultimately, our mindset creates our life.

When seemingly negative things happen, we can lament how unfair things are, or we can choose to allow each circumstance—be it challenge, success, or disappointment—to make us stronger, wiser, more knowledgeable, more skillful, more brave, and more loving. Life is full of choices, and what we make of them determines our experience. Recognizing that our life experience is a product of our perspective, approach, and decisions—our mindset—is what developing personal responsibility is all about.

In the book *The Big Leap*, psychologist Gay Hendricks points out that in relational conflict each entity (person, organization, country, etc.) owns 100 percent of the responsibility for resolving the conflict. (Yes, that adds up to 200 percent. Stay with me here.) He asserts that the fatal mistake is thinking that there is 100 percent responsibility to be divided up, because in that scenario, each entity has to be assigned some part of the 100 percent. And this assigning of blame is where the shit hits the fan. Because we end up lock-horned in this endless—hours, days, years, decades—bid for Biggest Victim status. We are better served when we stop trying to assign blame for our life situation to other people and events. Our experience of our life is 100 percent ours. We have little or no control over other people and events, but we can have 100 percent control over our perspective—our experience of those people and events.

A simple example of this is when we apologize and then add a "but" onto the end of it. "Everyone I know has a big but," as Pee-Wee Herman quipped with an eyeroll in the movie *Pee-Wee Herman's Great Adventure*. (The spelling, and his character's play on words, was intentional.) For example, *"I'm sorry that I shouted at you, but you shouldn't be so careless with other people's property."* Ouch. The "but you shouldn't be so careless" pretty much annihilates the apology. The message is: *I may have yelled and acted badly, but I acted badly only because you made me do so with your careless behavior. If you weren't such a careless jerk, I would never have been pulled from my pedestal of perfect behavior.* This kind of Big But—splitting up the blame pie so that we get the smallest slice—plays out in our lives in small and big ways, every day.

The more complex manifestations of Big But can be challenging and require us to be even more present and honest with ourselves. Years back, I had an eighteen-month period where the following happened: I got divorced, with four kids in the mix; I had to move out of our family home with my sons and I had seven weeks to find a new place to live; our family dog died; one son was getting bullied; and I had a large financial loss that threatened my ability to keep us in our new home. It was one of those "perfect storm" periods that many of us experience, when we stand seemingly alone, wet, and shivering in the eye of the tempest, shouting at the dark and punishing sky, *"Why me?!"*

A storm is an appropriate metaphor, because you and I know that storms don't happen to us, they simply happen. It's not personal. I'm not proud to admit that I spent a fair amount of my time during that period feeling as if things were happening *to me*, and feeling like a victim. I blamed my husband for the issues in our marriage; I blamed our divorce for killing our dog (I know that sounds weird, but he was really stressed by our split); I blamed the kids who were bullying my son; and I blamed my tax accountant for the financial fiasco that almost cost us our home. I was scared, exhausted, and sometimes feeling sorry for myself. Even once we understand personal responsibility, it's easy to get caught in that swirl and lose sight of what we know serves us.

Eventually, I was so run down that I got pneumonia; I received that as a wake-up call. My body was saying, *"Enough is enough, woman."* Over time, I took back 100 percent responsibility for my life experience. I rediscovered that owning my life experience was empowering and liberating. Our marriage had ended because we *both* contributed to poor communication and dysfunction. My dog died because he was sick. The best thing I could do for my son was to guide him through navigating bullies and staying true to himself, because bullies pop up in our lives well past childhood. There were signs along the way of the tax issue that I had chosen to ignore; in truth, I had stuck my head in the sand, hoping that the issues would go away and they didn't.

This change in perspective didn't mean that other people hadn't contributed to my perfect storm. It simply meant that I was able to choose how I perceive and respond to what happened in my life. Having a Big But (excuses) is most often a way of skirting personal responsibility; life just *is*; it's our railing against life events that's the real issue. The dark storm seems like the bad guy, but if we can turn our curiosity to it and dare to understand, it can teach us profound lessons, personally and relationally. In my story, the "storm" was a deeply challenging time during which I leaned into what was uncomfortable and learned a lot about Owning It.

A simple way to use *owning it* in your everyday life is to repeat this mantra to yourself whenever you find yourself sliding into the victim mentality trap: *"When things are working, I'm responsible. When things aren't working, I'm responsible."* In other words, we are 100 percent responsible for our life experience. Taking personal responsibility for your life experience is the first pillar we're exploring together because it's the only way to start moving forward.

As long as we're waiting for someone else to fix us; to love and care for us; to make our life better; and to make us feel attractive, whole, and worthy, then the next two pillars of self-worth and self-care aren't useful. What you'll discover, over time, is that personal responsibility is empowering and contains the potential to significantly improve your life experience.

Ownership Equals Empowerment

Personal responsibility is as essential to a healthy and joyful life experience as oxygen is to human life. It's fuel for the fire. Building the habit of personal responsibility hinges on asking ourselves good questions: *"Is this in my circle of concern or my circle of influence? How can I reframe this problem in the Creator Mindset, instead of the Victim Mindset? How can I own this messy situation in a way that empowers me?"*

Personal responsibility doesn't mean you're a one-(wo)man show. It takes a village, for sure. When I come down with pneumonia or break my arm, I seek the advice of my doctor. When I'm unhappy in my marriage and feeling stuck in my life, I seek out a therapist. When I'm struggling with my business, I turn to business coaches, trainers, brilliant colleagues, and mentors. When I'm struggling with parenting, I read books and talk to the best parents I know. The ingredient that remains the same in all of those scenarios is me and my choices—I am exercising my creator abilities in my circle of influence—creating my experience of life. We must own our life because we can't influence what isn't ours. By owning it—all of our experience—we now have placed ourselves squarely in the driver's seat. Which is empowering. Personal responsibility will change the entire weave and fabric of your life experience, in tiny and big ways that you'd never imagine. One big way that it serves us is that it builds up our self-worth.

CHAPTER 4:

THE SELF-WORTH PILLAR: YOU ARE ENOUGH

"You alone are enough. You have nothing to prove to anybody."

—MAYA ANGELOU

Many of us struggle, in ways big and small, in the business of everyday human life. I believe there are three main reasons: the first is our resistance; the second is our disconnection from the bigger part of ourselves, our spirit. The third is, as imperfect beings knocking around on this planet, we struggle with the common affliction of low self-worth.

Indeed, one of the deepest forms of suffering in our twenty-first century society is the pain of believing that "something is wrong" with ourselves. Feeling that we're continually falling short of worthiness is akin to breathing toxic gas. It makes it difficult to be truly intimate with others or at home in our bodies, our hearts, or our minds. Whether in the shape of chronic self-judgment, blaming others, depression, anxiety, or shame—feelings of deficiency prevent us from living and loving fully. As such, the second foundational pillar that will support your health, joy, and personal evolution is the pillar of your *self-worth*.

What Is Self-Worth?

Self-worth comes from loving and accepting who we are, regardless of our pant size, our occupation, our past, our net worth, or whether our kid is an "A" student or not. **Self-worth** is a sense of one's own intrinsic value or worth as a person. Self-worth is confidence we have in our unique expression of personhood and an unshakeable faith in ourselves. Confidence is not arrogance. Arrogance is most often an outward disguise for the low self-worth that lurks behind a self-assured mask. True confidence is grounded in a quiet humility that says, *"I am good enough and I like me."* As it's been said, "It's not what you are that is holding you back. It's what you think you are not." Said another way, building healthy self-worth doesn't require us to change who we are. Instead, it simply requires that we accept who we are, in this moment, in all our flawed majesty. We embrace that we're okay. However, as I'll continue to remind you throughout our time together, what's simple often isn't easy. This is especially true in the arena of our self-worth, as it's not something that we typically think about. Our self-worth exists off our radar.

The Unnamed Pain

Self-worth isn't on our radar because it is often discounted as a touchy-feely thing that mature, together, cool people don't need to waste their time with. This fallacy leads to self-worth not getting the attention it needs in our homes, schools, or in our culture-at-large. Our self-worth, individually and globally, is on the decline. This is our unnamed pain. We've bought into a culture where we're defined by our labels—successful, failure, attractive, ugly, smart, dumb, extrovert, introvert—instead of understanding that we're defined by something much bigger and more powerful than these rather unimportant and subjective labels.

The extreme culture change that's been ushered in by the information age, combined with our inability or refusal to face our unnamed pain, is eroding our sense of self. As one generation of people with low self-worth raises the next generation, the problem seeds and compounds itself.

Until we become serious about embracing our truth, we'll continue to feel restless and unhappy. Unfortunately, our poor self-worth affects more than we imagine. It affects our decisions, large and small. It affects who we choose to spend our time with, as we tend to choose friends and partners who reflect our self-worth. It affects how we run our job, our career, our business. It affects our parenting. It affects each interaction that we have.

When our self-worth is in full flower, we're coming from a place of enough-ness, of wholeness, of fullness, so we aren't looking for anything outside of ourselves to do anything for us or to fix anything. When our self-worth is wilted or damaged, we make choices and decisions based on trying to prove we're worthy, or trying to fill the void of our self-worth with outside approval. Sometimes, this approval-seeking becomes addictive, as in the case of technology.

Technology Travesty

The technology age has changed how we relate, do business, learn, travel, eat, and date. Personal technology devices have changed what we value. Our use of these devices has changed our economy and it has changed our world politics. Overnight, from an evolutionary standpoint, the technology age has created deep and far-reaching changes in almost every crevice of our daily lives. As with most things, there are pluses and minuses to this rapid transformation of our culture. Although there are many factors that contribute to our declining self-worth, science points to technology as a quiet yet formidable contributor. How is this so?

We've become dependent on constant validation from outside ourselves, in the form of social media—likes, Tweets, followers, and engagement. In the case of the Generation Z population, who has grown up with personal technology and social media, research shows that they actually feel anxious when their smartphone is not in hand. They're lost without the instant validation that social media provides, even though the majority of it comes from inconsequential sources. Research has revealed that most of us have three to five close friends—people with whom we have deep and trusting relationships—which means the majority of our hundreds or thousands of social media friends and followers are people we don't know well, if at all. This is what I mean by inconsequential. Meanwhile, there's an increasing sense that if you don't post it, it didn't happen. So we post and engage. A lot. When feedback happens that gives us pleasure, we get a dopamine hit. It chemically makes us feel good. And we want more of it.

Addiction is tied to dopamine. With personal technology devices and social media, we're being reprogrammed on a cellular level to require *constant* feedback from the dopamine reward system in order to feel good, to feel like we're enough. Social media addiction is a real thing; the result is that we become dependent on that device in our hand to make us feel wanted, included, liked, and worthy.

We used to get occasional validation from the three to five people whom we loved and trusted most, and most of our self-worth was implicit. Now we require continual validation from hundreds, thousands, of people who don't know us well and who often don't have our best interest at heart. Meanwhile, as we scroll through social media feeds, we're subconsciously comparing our real-life messy insides with other people's fictitious oh-so-perfect outsides. Yet, since dopamine is involved, we crave the flimsy, meaningless validation that we sometimes receive, and it begins to define our sense of self. This idea of continual, outwardly validated worth makes it hard for anyone to develop and maintain a healthy, balanced perception of their self-worth, even in the best of circumstances.

Adding insult to injury, we live in an age where many parents are addicted (alcohol, drugs, technology, work, social media, shopping) and staring at their phones; more and more kids are growing up feeling that subtle but insidious form of trauma called neglect. Because no one really sees them. Their parents are lost in their own search for validation. These children later find that regardless of what they add to their life as adults, their insides feel a bit broken; unseen and unseeable; a covert pain that they can't even name. It's no wonder that many of us struggle with self-worth issues to varying degrees. This low self-worth creates and reinforces our addictions, which then further lowers our self-worth because now we additionally feel badly about our addictions. Our self-worth is under attack from the powerful social and cultural forces around us.

This low self-worth manifests in many ways. One of the most disturbing is a high suicide rate, particularly among men. The millennial generation has the highest level of suicide in any generation in history. The number two cause of death among men and teenage boys under thirty-five—which includes millennials and Gen Z—is suicide. As I write this, I'm not sure what to say about this tragic statistical trend. This I do know: we have to get to the root of trauma and low self-worth.

The Fall of Self-Worth

How might we do that? What is the typical trajectory of self-worth, aside from technology? Even for folks that grow up in a fairly loving, stable home, self-worth is something that can slowly be worn away over time, without us even realizing it. Let's say that our life starts out pretty well. We're born healthy, our essential needs are met, and we're not living in fear. We all come into this physical existence packaged up with love, curiosity, and creativity— just burgeoning with self-expression. We're not concerned with what anyone else thinks about our self-expressive outfit, our loud laugh, our off-key singing voices, our crazy dance moves, or our unruly hair. We know how to play, create, and love without holding back. Joy is our natural state. We don't think of ourselves as anything less than 100 percent amazing.

Then, we get "socialized."

As we absorb ideas of who we are from the people around us—parents, family members, teachers, coaches, peers, neighbors—we replace many of our innate knowings with negative false beliefs about ourselves. Our young self is programmed by our environment. We have yet to understand that our sense of self cannot be given or taken away by others. It cannot be eroded or improved by anything in our childhood experience—"making" our parents happy, getting bad grades in school, "making" our parents unhappy, playing a varsity sport, winning the spelling bee, refusing to practice the piano, or not being accepted by the cool kids. But our identity as a powerful Creator is being socialized out of us, so we replace I-am-awesome with doubt, with fear, and with shame.

There are three paths that this takes us down:

1. We settle for the mediocrity of working hard to meet the expectations of our family, of our tribe, and of our culture—while on a constant search for what will finally make us feel happy and whole.

2. We escape our pain by numbing it with alcohol, drugs, sex, food, TV, internet, social media, shopping, or video games, which often leads to a cycle of addiction.

3. We continually jury-rig aspects of our outward appearance, persona, and achievements in order to gain the acceptance and accolades from others that we can't provide to ourselves.

The first path, mediocrity, leaves us feeling restless, invisible, and vaguely lonely and discontent. The second path of numbing the pain of our low self-worth has many difficult outcomes and inevitably increases our isolation and pain. Path number three of jury-rigging our feelings of enough-ness has many manifestations, and one is particularly insidious: our relentless pursuit of perfection. Chasing perfection is a way of continually running from fear. Our fear that we'll be found out. That the jury-rigged outward image of ourselves that's held in place by our low self-worth will be bared for the world to see. Elizabeth Gilbert wrote in her book *Big Magic*: "Perfection is fear in high-heeled shoes." Meaning, this jury-rigged socially accepted view of ourselves may *look* good, but it is fear masquerading as Put-Together.

The Myth of Perfection

Perfectionism and a healthy self-worth don't co-exist. Perfectionism requires a static and unmoving world; a perfectionist psyche can feel okay only if everything is completely reliable and controllable. This is, of course, impossible, as we live in a world based on flow and change. If you find yourself focusing on the philosophies and practices in this book with grim determination and perfectionism, understand this: the flow inside you has evaporated, and you're now working against wholeness and self-worth. Wholeness includes the entirety of our existence—peace and turmoil, grace and clumsiness, competence and incompetence, winning and losing, clarity and confusion, success and failure. Perfectionism, on the other hand, only accepts half of our existence—those parts that will maintain our rigid image of Put-Together—peace, grace, competence, good looks, winning, clarity, and success. Perfectionism is analogous to a tiny Pac-Man who methodically devours us from the inside.

I see my friends, clients, and students struggle with this every day. I also know this one well, as I lived it for decades. I remember sitting in my therapist's office about seven years ago, feeling like a fraud in my put-together white-picket-fence life, feeling like I wanted to crawl out of my skin, wondering who I really was. I looked her straight in the eye and said, "I want to become a ball dropper." As someone who most always kept all the balls in the air and worked to excel at everything I did, including the stuff I didn't want to do and the stuff that didn't matter (?!?!), I wanted to know how it would feel to *not* be that. I wanted to know what it would feel like to uncover and live the life that resonated with me, instead of the life that I imagined was expected of me. I had a hunch that my pursuit of perfection was a big part of my discontent; I had come to the point where I imagined that I certainly couldn't feel *worse* by allowing myself to drop balls and see how it went. I wanted to look at myself in the mirror and see who was there, beneath the continual striving for perfection. I wanted to do a trust fall into the arms of my authentic self.

This is a case of be careful what you ask for, and a reminder that we often don't know what we want or what form we want it in. For me, I was launched into a period of intense self-questioning, divorce, and moving. This then required that I become the main steward of a home, my business, family finances, and the many daily logistics of parenting. Those were the four scariest-feeling, most humbling years of my life—and I wouldn't change a thing. Because I like the other side, and I like myself. Do I still sometimes find myself with one foot sliding into that pair of high-heeled perfection? I do. But I'm more aware now. I know that those shoes may look great on me, but they hurt my feet, knees, and back. I know that about 90 percent of the time, they don't fit with who I Am, and that the reason I've been subconsciously wiggling my foot into one again is because I'm afraid. Afraid of success or afraid of failure. Afraid of loving or afraid of being alone. Afraid of being seen or afraid of not being seen. And that's okay. I don't need to be perfect in my release of perfection. I get incrementally more aware, and better at stopping the madness before it gets started.

Perfection is a tricky addiction because our culture not only accepts it, unlike taboo addictions such as drugs or sex, but it actually encourages it. Globally, the beauty and diet industries were worth over $700 billion in 2017. One could argue that a portion of that market is the result of people pursuing better health, and this is true. However, the vast majority of this sector markets to people—particularly women—with the message that they're not enough. This marketing encourages our feelings of low self-worth, while promising to fix it. It doesn't, of course. Even if we do lose the ten pounds of belly fat in twenty days; create unvaried, pore-less skin; or magically grow hair on our bald spot, we still feel vaguely unhappy and not-enough. We're simply a skinnier, air-brushed-looking, or hairier version of our unhappy self. Meanwhile, a lack of self-worth, stress, and exhaustion are lapping at the edges of our sanity, threatening to pull the whole façade down, leaving our naked, imperfect self for the whole world to see.

Rather than wait for the breakdown, I suggest you start to bring the pursuit of perfection into your awareness and feel out if that's a tripping point for you. Maybe yes, maybe no. If yes, start by softening the edges as you build your self-worth. Start by learning to resonate with your truth.

The Truth of You

The truth of you is that you can't be defined by anything outside of yourself—possessions, status, fame, job, appearance, roles—none of that is "you." You're a good parent? . . . That's not you. You're a bad parent? . . . That's not you. You have a yacht? . . . That's not you. You're homeless? . . . That's not you. You created a new technology? . . . That's not you. You're a drug addict? . . . That's not you.

The real you is much more than all the labels that the mind adheres to. The real you is not defined by any label, positive or negative. You are that unique and scrumptious blending of body, mind, and spirit that you showed up with on day one. You're defined by the heart and spirit that you embody, live, and express in your everyday messy and imperfect life. We're all perfectly imperfect. To think anything less is as silly as a beach thinking its sand is too uneven, its waves too loud, or its water too cold. Says who? I have yet to meet a beach I didn't like. Sure, I enjoy some more than others, but they're all amazing in their own way. You're the only you there has ever been, the only you there is, and the only you that ever will be. You may not be enough for everyone, but what matters is that you're enough for yourself.

The truth of our self-worth can take time and effort to lean into, and that journey can sometimes be uncomfortable. We do what we can to heal our trauma; and we set out to remember how truly amazing we are by peeling back the layers of socialized self-beliefs to get back to what we knew in the beginning—that we *are* love and joy embodied. When we truly love and honor ourselves—recognizing and embracing the worth that's been there all along—everything else in our life becomes easier, healthier, and more joyful. We move along a continuum of healing, enjoying deeper connection to those around us.

You Don't Know What You Don't Know

Middle school was a challenging time for me, as it was for many. In seventh grade, in addition to typical teenage struggles—having a serious disconnect with my dad, feeling lonely and misunderstood at home, struggling with self-image around my increasingly gangly and awkward body, and trying to socially fit in—my grades started to slide. My mom couldn't make sense of it because I'd always been a kid who enjoyed school. Thankfully, one of the teachers mentioned to my mom that she'd noticed me squinting to look at the blackboard. Mom took me to an eye doctor, who told her there was nothing wrong with my eyes, and that I was probably doing this for attention. My mom didn't buy that.

The next eye doctor found that my vision was impaired. He prescribed corrective lenses and we ordered some glasses. A few weeks later, my mom and I drove to pick them up and have them fitted. When we got into the car and started the drive home, I was stunned into silence, watching in amazement as a new world slid by my window. I could see everything—every exquisite detail and every contrast of color. Strands of hair on the woman on the crosswalk. The individual birds feeding on the park grass. The plaid on a man's shirt stood out in sharp detail. The cat licking his paw on the sidewalk had a buckle on his collar. And the trees. Oh, the trees. "Mom, I can see all the leaves on the trees! Can you see that?" I asked. She assured me she could. I had assumed that everyone saw trees as giant lollipops with brown sticks and a green circle of candy. I could see all the beauty and detail of our little blue-collar Maine town and couldn't imagine ever getting tired of taking in all that I'd missed.

Finally seeing your self-worth is just like that. When you aren't familiar with the feeling of being centered in who you are; of feeling accepting and loving of yourself; and not feeling the need to prove yourself to anyone, including yourself, you simply have no frame of reference for what it would feel like to have self-worth. It's hard to imagine the energy, productivity, and creativity that you'll have when you take back the energy expended on constantly evading, placating, or numbing a low self-worth. You can't imagine a tree with leaves if you've never seen one.

The difference between my middle-school vision issues and our self-worth is that we can't simply put on self-worth glasses to suddenly see ourselves in all of our inherent amazingness. Self-worth starts slowly and then grows over time, coming up like a small green hint of life from an acorn in the sun, growing into a sturdy oak tree of self-worth in the light of your awareness. Over time, it will grow into a bigger and bigger oak tree—a nature-created pillar—with a solid trunk and many branches and leaves. It might experience a challenge now and then—a storm, an insect infestation, a drought—but it has resources for recovery. Self-worth and oak trees can grow deep root systems, gaining strength and longevity for the long haul.

First Step Toward Wholeness

Imagine a world where everyone's self-worth increased even a measly 25 percent. How would our experience be if all of humanity's enough-ness was no longer threatened by other people's opinions, gender identity, sexual expression, skin color, nationality, religion, talents, formal education accomplishments, traditions, job, income, or self-expression? If our self-worth no longer needed us to label and judge others in order to help us feel better about ourselves, our choices, and our life experience? This would be a powerful move toward a more sane world.

No one can give us a seven-step program for improving our self-worth. What we can do is take the first step, which is almost always the same in any area where we desire a shift—our amigo *awareness*. We become aware of the ways we see ourselves as not-enough. Although this can feel scary and make us feel vulnerable, our self-worth can't heal when our fear and pain are left deep inside us, where we buried them in our youth, and where they continued to stockpile as we aged. The light of our awareness and self-compassion will start the healing process—in the same way that the sun brings the first hint of an oak tree out of the hard shell of an acorn. The good news is that developing our self-worth is less often about analyzing our wounds and neuroses and more often about generating and accepting self-love. It's about knowing that the people who hurt us and told us we weren't enough were likely hurting and feeling unworthy themselves. Hurt people hurt people.

At a certain point, having seen why a pattern developed (*"My ex-wife always belittled me in front of others"*) and the effect it has had on our self-worth *("I adored her, gave her power over me, and started believing what she said"),* actual change in our self-worth occurs because of a decision on our part: the decision to heal. It ultimately doesn't matter so much *why* we became angry, reckless, or defensive. It's a good data point, and is part of awareness, but it's not the part that heals us. Ultimately, it's coming home to ourselves that heals us. As such, the rest of the journey is individual and varies widely. Some folks work with a psychologist or counselor; some join a twelve-step program; others get involved with a spiritual group; while some journal, read, meditate, and reflect on their own. There are many paths that lead to our positive self-worth, and they all begin with awareness.

I invite you to let this discussion marinate in your mind, and to maybe revisit it after reading Chapter 8. You see, your true self-worth is owned wholly by you, and it's part of your birthright. Your sense of self—as love and joy—and your positive self-worth lies within you. With time and attention, we can learn to not torture ourselves anymore, to make friends with ourselves, and to love ourselves. Loving and caring for ourselves takes many forms, and the next chapter will illuminate how we can get started.

CHAPTER 5:

THE SELF-CARE PILLAR: FILL YOUR CUP

"Self-care is not selfish. You cannot serve from an empty vessel."

—ELEANOR BROWNN

I looked at the picture again and reread the article to be sure I didn't miss anything. It was an article about a mother of three who was undergoing chemotherapy and radiation for an aggressive form of cancer, and the topic thread was how heroic she was for not missing a beat when it came to caring for her husband and children. My two sons were under five years old and my two stepdaughters were teenagers, and I was feeling wrung-out a fair amount of the time. But this other mother? She attended PTA meetings, went to all of their sporting events, helped fill out college applications, made family meals, and drove her teenage children everywhere. (If you are a parent of teenagers, you know that driving is a part-time job all on its own.)

The article exalted her sacrifice of putting her health challenge on the back burner in order to be a "good mother," and praised how she made sure that her kids didn't feel the impact of her grave illness. The article painted this mom as a role model for other mothers, with her selfless attention to her family, even as she struggled to keep the nausea from her chemo treatments at bay.

I felt sad reading the article—sad that we're fed this misaligned virtue as something to strive for in our media, marketing, and our culture. Sad that to be a "good mom" means to wring every last drop of ourselves out in order to make sure that no one else is inconvenienced by our illness, our challenging day, our migraine. This expectation seems imbalanced and unhealthy.

We all—men, women, moms, dads, teenagers, seniors—need self-care. I'm talking here about true self-care, which is a form of self-love. Yet, modern messaging around self-care is confusing at best and damaging at worst. Despite advertising that showers us with products and destinations that espouse to promote self-care, the unspoken message in our culture is that we should care for everyone else first, especially as women. For men and women, especially during parenting years, the message is that our self-care can't get in the way of anyone else's convenience, otherwise it's selfish. Yet when our cups are empty, we have nothing to share with others. Let's unpack that irony into something more workable and supportive of everyday life and health.

Self-care is care provided for you, by you. It's about identifying your individual needs for well-being and taking steps to meet them, on a daily basis, acting from a place of support and love. This self-care deeply affects our attitude about life experiences while creating consistent, gentle support that helps us express and live the most vibrant and satisfied version of ourselves. As wonderful as this sounds, it's important to make a subtle distinction: self-care is different from self-indulgence. Self-care can sometimes feel not-fun in the moment, such as when we drag our ass out of bed on a cold winter morning to get to our spin class.

You see, self-care supports us in maintaining our health, in living more joyfully, and in feeling more vibrant in our daily life—with an eye to the long haul. Prioritizing self-care isn't selfish; it's absolutely essential for everything else in our lives to be amazing. It supports us on all levels, BodyMindSpirit, and helps us to be the most joyful and effective we can be in all our roles: as a parent, friend, partner, daughter, son, colleague, teacher, employee, board member, employer, or student. We need to radically change our relationship with self-care.

"I don't have time for self-care! I don't think you understand how busy I am."

This is what we tell ourselves. Unfortunately, our well-being hangs in the balance. We either prioritize and create time now or we often end up having to make time down the road for rehab, job troubles, therapy, a mental breakdown, a divorce, health issues, or stressed-out kids who don't know how to care for themselves. I'm not exaggerating here just to make my point. I see the collateral damage of people's lack of self-care each day in my work, and I've seen it looking back at myself in the mirror as well. Ultimately, if we can't see our way to sending this love and compassion our way, the rest of the ideas in this book are simply theory. I've heard every excuse out there for why we don't have time for self-care. It's interesting to watch how hard people will push back on this one. I've watched it over and over in my clinical and integrative health practice, with my friends and family, with my corporate clients, and at speaking events.

Cultivating our self-care mojo is one area where our growing personal responsibility *("If I want to feel happier, healthier, and more joyful, I need to do something about it")* and our deepening awareness of our self-worth *("I'm an amazing spirit in human form and the evolution of me and of the world requires me to be at my best. I'm worth it")* give us a big leg up. Working with those first two pillars of personal responsibility and self-worth helps us clear out the years of programming that tells us self-care is selfish and that we must sacrifice our needs, at all times, for the good of others.

Creating Self-Care Habits

Self-care looks different for different people. A client of mine who owns and runs a thriving company faithfully goes to a boxing class each Tuesday night after work with her teenage daughter. It's a delicious combo of sass-building strength, mother-daughter time, and some serious stress release. It helps her feel calm and connected to herself. All of these things feel good to her, making the class a foundational part of her self-care. Boxing isn't for me; walking solo and barefoot in nature is my thing. Movement, solitude, and a deep connection to nature releases stress from the fabric of my being and helps me feel calmer and more connected to myself. Two different people, two different choices in the self-care department.

What works for you? I invite you to look through the following list of some of the most common self-care practices. Some of them, such as nourishing food, hydrating, and protecting our sleep, are important for all of us— while some are individual, like boxing vs. walking barefoot in nature. This list is not exhaustive; my hope is that it will get your creative juices flowing, helping you to craft your specific list. Remember, our life experience is created in large part by our habits; so the question to ask yourself now is: *which micromovement(s) am I able and willing to make first?*

Forms of self-care include:

Eating health-building food

Hydrating (drinking plenty of water)

Protecting sleep time and quality

Scheduling recharge time (listening to music, knitting, coloring, gardening)

Moving (including exercise like walking or hiking in nature)

Enjoying a sporting event with friends

Meditating

Dancing

Practicing yoga

Playing golf with friends

Breathing deeply

Nurturing positive social connections

Creating regular off-the-grid time

Sitting doing nothing, or taking a nap

Setting and maintaining healthy boundaries

There are many ways to nurture ourselves. What's important, as you change your relationship with self-care, is that you're mindful of building a framework for success. Life is guaranteed to have ups and downs, and it's helpful to focus on ways to make your self-care framework as unshakeable as possible, so you can reap the benefits when you need them the most. Let's explore five tenets that will help.

Tenet 1: Release Old, Tired Beliefs

Neither guilt nor martyr-hood have a place in self-care. A belief system that dictates that we should be constantly in service to others and continually productive, and that a clean house should come before a hot bath, isn't serving our health on any level—body, mind, or spirit. This compulsion that some of us have to be productive every moment of the day is total BS fed to us by our keep-up culture: *If you're not doing something, you're probably not very important or interesting.* There's no prize at the end of our lives for chronically putting ourselves last. Looking at the big picture, our family and friends will love us for who we are, not for what we do for them.

It's critical that we find out what relaxes us, nourishes our BodyMind-Spirit, and allows us to rest and repair—and to intentionally do more of that. I suggest a new mantra such as: *"I'm loving this _____ [time in the garden, hike, quiet reading time], and I also know it's supporting every other aspect of my life."* When you first say this, you may well feel like a fraud or a liar. Moreover, change is hard, especially when it comes to changing our habits of mind. Keep trying, keep coming back to the mantra, and the repetition will eventually create a belief. Like any new habit, repeating this mantra to ourselves and making room in our lives for self-care can feel weird. Weird is not synonymous with bad or wrong. Weird is more often synonymous with different, unfamiliar, wonky, or novel. I encourage you to give a nod to this wonky feeling and carry on with your self-care and your mantra.

Tenet 2: Consistency

Although getting a monthly massage can be a fabulous and highly recommended activity, it doesn't provide the everyday support that we need. A massage is an event, not a habit. Self-care that's a mindful part of our everyday life gets us the biggest bang for our buck. My sister Leslie, for example, is clockwork-consistent with her yoga. Even when she's traveling, her yoga practice comes with her; it's a habit.

Another family example that I often share with students outlines the idea of consistency well. For as long as I can remember, each morning and evening, my mother sits in a chair and drinks tea. That's it. No reading, no phone, no conversation. Just a woman and her warm mug. I believe that this practice is loosely meditational for my mom. She's simply relaxing, quieting her mind, and putting herself first—and the mug-o-tea is her version of a meditation focus point instead of breath.

As I got older, I realized that when I drank tea, it helped me feel relaxed and cared for, even when I served it to myself. This makes sense because I had years of conditioning, watching my mom relax with tea, telling me that this is what tea does for someone. So I've started having tea with me whenever I'm in the car, and often while I'm working, to help me feel less stressed. I had to do the planning to support my new portable self-care habit. It required that I stock teas I enjoy, have mugs that feel nice in my hand, and carry a travel mug. My tea self-care is a small and doable habit that happens each day, multiple times. It helps me feel cared for; I relish that first whiff of Egyptian Licorice, Green, Lemon Ginger, or Indian Chai Spice. I'm serving myself some self-love in a cup, and I'm hydrating too. Tea might not be your thing, but I imagine you get the idea: consistency is key.

Tenet 3: Self-Care Comes First

When we're stressed or overburdened, self-care needs to come first. Typically, however, self-care is the first thing to go under stress and, paradoxically, that self-neglect makes us feel even more stressed and overburdened. This is a tricky one, I know. Often, when we feel stressed out or overburdened, a key aspect of that feeling is thinking that we don't have enough time to get things done. So, it would make sense that we would find time by cutting back on, or eliminating, our self-care. We cut back on sleep, we skip exercise, lean into easy packaged and fast foods, blow off our yoga and meditation. I know the drill, I've done it myself; I also know that the time that we "gain" when doing this is a smoke-and-mirrors situation. It works out okay-ish for one or two days, and then it catches up with us.

The bank account of our health and sanity operates on a give-and-take maintaining of balance. You can only make so many withdrawals without making some deposits. If we're growing our checking account with deposits, then we can write checks, pay bills, and grab some cash from the ATM. If we're not making deposits, eventually we can't make any more withdrawals. In the world of your well-being, deposits (self-care) and withdrawals (work, caring for others, household tasks) need to have a good balance in the same way that they do in your checking account.

Again, I know this can be hard when the pressure's on. I suggest never skimping on sleep, which we'll talk more about when we discuss honoring the body. Studies show that if we're getting less than seven and a half hours of sleep per night, then we're sleep deprived, regardless of our insistence that we can easily get by on only four to six hours of sleep. The amount of important healing and maintenance work that our body and mind does during sleep is staggering. Further, we don't think as clearly when we're sleep-deprived; we also tend to be more moody, negative, and volatile. Our willpower is also significantly diminished by lack of sleep. None of these byproducts of chronic sleep deprivation are improving our life experience. Although we feel as if we have more time, it's less productive time and we tend to be less creative and make more mistakes. Sleep is a good one to schedule, each night, like it's the most important meeting of your day.

Tenet 4: Create Healthy Boundaries

Creating healthy boundaries is not only an integral part of self-care, it's empowering. By recognizing the need to set and enforce limits, we protect our self-esteem, maintain self-respect, and enjoy healthy relationships.

Unfortunately, boundary setting is a skill that few of us are taught. Although creating and maintaining boundaries is sometimes hard, it's important. Many folks struggle with this concept of boundaries, saying that it feels mean or selfish, that the word *boundaries* sounds like the word *walls,* and that they're not interested in being that person. I misunderstood boundaries too and have come to understand that boundaries are different than barriers. **Boundaries** mean being clear with what is okay—and not okay— for us. Being clear about our boundaries helps us honor ourselves and honor others while supporting ourselves in staying whole. No one else can see or know what kind of space and time we need to stay happy, focused, and sane. Often, we aren't even clear about what we need ourselves, and we all have different boundary needs. For instance, I do well with a fair amount of time in solitude, and some people need little or none at all.

Because boundary needs vary widely from person to person, an important first step in creating healthy boundaries is one of our Three Amigos:

awareness. Bring awareness to your life situations and take notice. Where do you feel edgy? Where are you playing the martyr? Where do you feel resentful? Where do you feel violated or uncomfortable? Once you become aware, you can start to create boundaries in that area, while being honest and kind to those who might be affected by those new boundaries. Building better boundaries might look like this:

- Bring awareness to your everyday life and uncover where you feel short-changed or chronically uncomfortable. Where are you giving away your time? Who are you spending your time with?

- Tune in to those shortchanged feelings and sit with them. What are you tolerating? Where is a boundary missing?

- Give yourself permission to create the boundaries you need, while honoring the feelings of others. Keep communication open, honest, and kind. Be direct and compassionate, with others and with yourself.

- Stay alert.

Once you've set a boundary, you need to protect it and be aware of changing needs you may have. We're constantly in flux, and our needs, desires, and outlooks change.

Remember that boundaries aren't just a sign of a healthy relationship; they're an act of self-respect that helps to buoy our self-worth. Creating firm, loving boundaries may also lead us to consider our relationship choices—those with whom we choose to share the bond of friendship and romantic love. In close relationships, we're influenced by the other person, so it serves us to be mindful about who we're hanging out with and to be aware of their influence. We're well-served to be selective about who we spend a lot of time with and to create boundaries that allow us to be our most aligned and loving selves. It matters more than most of us imagine. When we find that a person is hard for us in a way that doesn't support us, it's important to (gently, kindly) set boundaries. Whether we're on the side of creating boundaries or on the side of someone setting boundaries toward us, we don't have to take it personally when things cool off or come to an end.

Sometimes we even need space from the people that we really dig. At the end of my day, I often feel as if I'd give a million bucks to simply lie down and relax for a bit; this became especially true after my divorce. I had a conversation with my two sons and instituted Mom Time. Mom Time means that each night, I say goodnight to my kids, go into my bedroom and shut the door, and get into bed with a heating pad for my back and a good book. I enjoy the warmth on my back, the fresh air and night sounds coming in through my window, the tranquility, and my book. It's twenty minutes of heaven to wrap up my day, and my teenage kids know that this time is important to me. I'm off-duty and they don't bother me unless it truly can't wait. Twenty minutes may not sound like much, but because it's every night, that adds up to two hours and twenty minutes of self-care a week, just from this one habit. Remember that frequency and consistency are where we reap the most benefits from our self-care habits. Creating Mom Time involved a period of setting boundaries, with honesty and kindness, and helping my kids understand that I needed this quiet time to be the best possible version of myself so that I could be a more present and patient mom. Not only does it get me what I need, but it also teaches my kids how to respect the needs of others *and* tees them up to protect their own boundaries. Important stuff.

Tenet 5: Self-Care Feels Caring

A self-care subtlety that's important, and often missed, is that true self-care feels caring. These activities that we've discussed all have the ability to show ourselves that we love ourselves and are willing to support ourselves. However, our inner approach is critical. If we're doggedly pushing ourselves to do exercise that we hate doing, it's no longer true self-care. If we're doing yoga while we mentally check off all the things that need to get done today, we're not absorbing the full benefits of yoga. The self-care act is important, but our internal approach to that self-care is equally important. Our self-care practices must be done with an attitude of love and support to truly be self-care. And I have a good, messy story to illustrate my point.

In February 2015, I was a year and half past my official divorce and still deeply enmeshed in emotionally processing my life, my choices, and the question of who I was. Many of my relationships were changing as "couple friends" fell away. I was grappling with trying to be the best, most mindful single parent I could be, running a household on my own, growing and running a business, and trying to stay whole. These certainly aren't novel or unusual endeavors, but I was going through change and felt overwhelmed. To say that I was wound a bit tight would be an understatement. I worked hard to maintain self-care with exercise, yoga, health-building food, juicing, whole-food supplements, and frequent contact with friends and family. I also told myself I had a meditation practice, but it definitely wasn't consistent.

I was part-way through a year-long entrepreneurship training and was heading to a five-day training intensive in British Columbia, which is a long haul from Boston, especially during a snow storm that turned my seven-hour travel day into a twenty-three-hour travel day. I managed to extract myself from parenting, business, and household responsibilities for a whole week and set off for the lovely retreat center with delicious food and serene surroundings I'd seen online. However, I quickly learned that this was definitely an *intense*-ive. Our training started at 7:30 am every day and lasted until between 10:00 pm and 1:00 am; it was boot camp. I was pretty run-down when I left Boston for the training, and the long travel day added insult to injury. After a couple of days of this training schedule, although I was finding value in the training, I was worn pretty thin.

We started each day with a short thirty-minute yoga class with a top-notch instructor and guide, whom I will remember for life, named Jennifer. At the end of yoga class on day three, we were all in corpse pose, letting our bodies melt into the floor. As Jennifer walked around the room quietly talking and adjusting our poses, she said, "Maybe today is the day the war stops." Everything in me went still for a second or two, and then tears started *pouring* down my face. I waited for it to pass. It didn't. I rolled onto my side and into a fetal position, trying to cuddle myself into a calmer state so as not to disturb the forty business owners who lay on mats around me. People were starting to lift their heads and glance over to see what the fuss was about. As Jennifer passed by me, she stooped down and gently put a hand on my shoulder for a few seconds and then kept walking. That was it. The floodgates fully opened and I was audibly weeping while I blindly gathered my bag to hustle out the door. To outside and solitude and fresh air—surely that would calm me.

It didn't.

No matter what I did, I couldn't stop whatever had come unhinged inside me. I had no idea why that statement, "Maybe today is the day the war stops," had triggered such a response in me. I sobbed for hours while trying various tactics to calm myself down—standing in a frigid brook barefoot, deep breathing, a hot shower—but something needed to move through me, and it apparently wasn't timing itself around my business-training schedule. I felt like I was having a mental breakdown. In the second hot shower, my breathing finally started to slow down.

As I dried off and peered at my puffy, blotched face in the mirror, I had this out-of-body feeling of truly seeing myself. Not my image in the mirror, but Myself—the me who was suffocating under all the effort. I got dressed, gathered my training materials, and headed back out the door, dry-eyed, exhausted, and, somehow, a bit lighter. What I figured out through this inconvenient mini-breakdown was that throughout the year and a half since my divorce, when I'd been trying so hard to juggle so many responsibilities and navigate all the emotional pain that gets unleashed when a marriage ends, I had let all the *care* slip out of my self-care. I was doing "all the right things" to care for myself, but it had all become driven and pressured, little more than a punch-list of to-dos that the Vibrant Living Advocate does "to be healthy." It took this mini-breakdown for me to understand that it's our approach to self-care that's healing, more so than the mode of self-care. Therefore, if it applies, I hope today is the day you can stop the war against yourself. Please remember: self-care feels caring.

Getting Started

I invite you to choose one habit from the self-care list you crafted a few pages ago, that isn't part of your current self-care initiative, and commit to it for a month. The month-long period accomplishes two things: one, it gives you ample time to decide if you feel good with this habit added to your life; and two, since it takes twenty-one to sixty-six days to create a new habit, you've already laid the groundwork for the new neural pathways that will put your self-care on automatic.

For example, let's say you decide your food choices could use some sprucing up. Start with one meal and simply commit to having a health-building breakfast, lunch, or dinner each day for twenty-eight days. If you're not sure where to start, breakfast typically gets us the most bang for our buck. Next, you set yourself up for success with some planning. You decide on a few breakfasts that you'll rotate during the week. You stock all needed items in your kitchen and do any pre-prep. Then you decide how much, if any, extra time you need in the morning. If these are grab-n-go breakfasts, then that's zero minutes earlier that you need to get up. If you've decided to not only eat a health-building breakfast but also use it as a time to relax, you pad your morning schedule by twenty minutes and maybe make a hot breakfast and sit down and eat it to some relaxing music. This might sound like a lot of hoopla, but that's only because it's something new. After one to two months, this nurturing self-care will be part of your lifestyle, such as brushing your teeth or taking a shower.

I encourage you to have fun with this—and to be kind and gentle with yourself. Joyfully experiment with your self-care. Above all, create a self-care framework that feels good for you and works in your life. Try different things and put some thought into what will nourish your whole being. I encourage you to allow your self-care to be out in the open—with the people you live with, and with your inner circle of friends—and not something you squeeze in when no one's looking. Own your choices and feel good about sharing the power of your self-care with others. It might be just the permission they need to start practicing their own self-care. By filling your cup, you support others in filling theirs, as well. Your BodyMindSpirit health, as well as the health of our culture, depends on it.

Our self-care, self-worth, and personal responsibility pillars are essential to unlocking our potential for health and joy. Putting some time, thought, and effort into building these pillars for yourself is supportive on its own and helps you dance with the ideas that we'll cover in Part Two. Please know, however, that none of us has perfect pillars. Every aspect of our health journey co-creates and intermingles. Self-care, self-worth, and personal responsibility are all pillars unto themselves; they also further strengthen each other. For instance, self-care helps nurture our self-worth; and when people feel worthy, they're more likely to practice self-care. I invite you to enjoy the journey. This is not a stepped program but is instead an adventure that will look different for every reader of this book. And exploring the ways to honor our body and create physical health is on deck next.

PART TWO

JOYFUL HEART:
YOUR BODYMINDSPIRIT EVOLUTION

Each of us has the honor of being the sole steward of our mysterious, complex, and intricately powerful BodyMindSpirit. There is a distinct reason why I use the term **BodyMindSpirit** with our three aspects fused into one word. We are all that, and our health and joy—or lack thereof—is a result of their individual balance and of the interbalance of the three. The more I learn and experience, the more I find it difficult to separate our body, mind, and spirit aspects. They're intimately intertwined and synergistically affect one another and the world around them. Take a three-legged stool—it's impossible to say which of the legs is the most important. If one of the legs is weak or damaged, it creates stress on the other legs when the stool is sat upon. If one or two of the legs are too short, the sitter falls off.

Similarly, the body, mind, and spirit aspects of our being each affect and instruct one another. It's important to understand as you embark on these next three chapters, that though the body, mind, and spirit are presented in separate chapters, they're fundamentally one entity. Each of these three aspects of our wholeness must be paid attention to, honored, and healed where necessary if we're going experience more health and joy as part of our daily lives. Here's a story about my first client, which I think will show you what I'm talking about.

Jess was a lovely young schoolteacher who came to her appointments accompanied by her supportive, devoted husband. Jess rarely felt well and missed many work days due to her vast array of symptoms. She had a staggering list of food sensitivities, which most often points to a condition called leaky gut. This, combined with other information in her vigorous intake process, pointed to yeast overgrowth in her intestines, along with adrenal fatigue, as primary healing barriers to her dis-ease.

Why do I use the term *dis-ease*? Most of what we call disease, such as heart disease, diabetes, cancer, hypothyroid, acid reflux, or auto-immunity, is due to **dis-ease** in the human organism. We tend to think of disease as a prognosis, as the body deceiving us—a label of brokenness that we own. It's not. The development of disease is largely outside of our understanding; it's not our fault, and it doesn't define us. When I'm working with folks who are navigating a cancer challenge, I encourage them not to think of themselves as "a cancer patient," as this begets associating our identity with cancer. I suggest they instead think of themselves as a person who's navigating a cancer challenge. I also encourage people to say, *"I'm healing from* ____," instead of *"I have* ____*"* or *"I'm sick with* ____*."* It's a good idea to tell the fifty trillion cells that are listening in on our every thought that we're healing from something instead of that we're sick with it. In navigating whatever challenges come to our BodyMindSpirit, we must address ourselves as a whole in order to achieve true health, healing, and joy.

Okay, back to Jess. One important thing I learned in my clinical training is that the right thing, in the wrong order, is the wrong thing. This meant for Jess that, regardless of the fact that her adrenals were waving a white flag for attention, her digestion and absorption had to come first, starting with the yeast overgrowth in her intestinal tract. Hippocrates taught that, "All disease begins in the gut," and this is true the majority of the time. Having lived through my own battle with intestinal yeast—and having watched my father lose his battle with his, which had become systemic—I knew this journey professionally and personally. Jess and I worked together for several months, doing the right things in the right order physically, but Jess's health wasn't coming into balance. She had small windows of improvement and then dramatic dips.

Now, this was my first case out of grad school. I hadn't yet learned that I can't do the healing work *for* people—that's up to them and their Body-MindSpirit's healing faculties. Not knowing this yet, I stressed about Jess's health much more than was healthy for me. I was also feeling insecure and questioning whether I was doing the right things for her, because my only clinical experience had been in school and working with friends and family.

After a period of several months, during which Jess experienced intermittent healing, my intuition told me that there was something deeper and more personal at work here. I asked her if she'd be open to talking to a psychologist before continuing our work together; I hooked her up with a well-respected practitioner and let them get to work. The short story is that Jess, through excellent counseling, uncovered that although she was married to a wonderful man, she was gay. First, the simple act of empathy—in this case from a psychologist—directly improves our physiology. Second, once she recognized and embraced her true sexual orientation through some hard internal and external work, she began living her life more authentically. Ultimately, she healed. The work we'd started together began to gain momentum because of the healing in her mind. Yes, her physical aspect (her body) had some issues, but her mind aspect was struggling mightily. Jess's complex, beautiful Body-MindSpirit wasn't going to heal with simple attention to yeast, adrenals, and digestion. The life she was living wasn't aligned with who she was.

You see it turns out that we're not a victim of our heredity, or of our dis-ease. Each day, in many ways, we have the opportunity to be the master of our genetic activity—of our health and longevity. There's a growing body of research that supports integrated healing, and I've experienced the power of whole-person healing time and again in my work, and in my own life. It turns out that our idea that the genes we're born with determine our health and longevity wasn't the whole truth. The fate of our cells, and of the genetic code that's housed within them, lies in the *environment* in which those cells live—the environment of the cell is the trigger for genetic activity. That environment includes our thoughts, beliefs, and mental struggles.

This is the science of epigenetics, and the groundbreaking work of stem cell biologist Bruce Lipton has instructed my approach to healing and wellness in deep and profound ways. Food, exercise, sleep, stress, our thoughts, our beliefs, and our alignment with our spirit aspect all affect the expression of our DNA.

"Wait just a minute. You're telling me that thoughts and beliefs affect my physical health? They affect my DNA?! Surely you jest."

As alluded to in Jess's story, our thoughts, beliefs, and alignment with our true self are simply perceptions and interpretations of our life experience, which contribute to the internal environment of our body much as our blood chemistry does. There's a large and growing body of research that shows that these aspects of us are, indeed, part of the environment that our cells live in, and they affect our DNA. This puts us much more in the creator seat than in the victim seat in regards to our health and longevity, which is terrific news.

Our well-being is an intricate web of connections among the vast array of physiological aspects of our body, the clarity and use of our complex mind, and our connection to spirit. If one aspect is suffering, they all suffer and contribute to our health and life experience negatively. Further, sometimes things go amuck without any apparent cause. We're organisms, not machines. But we have much more influence than most of us imagine. If we more intentionally tend our expression of body, mind, spirit, each becomes more healthy on its own while also influencing the others, creating a self-actualizing, virtuous cycle. That cycle is what we're considering and exploring in Part Two. Let's get started with your beautiful body.

CHAPTER 6:

HONOR YOUR BODY

"Take care of your body. It's the only place you have to live."

—JIM ROHN

Getting Under the Hood

When I was twenty-two years old and had just graduated college with my shiny new bachelor's degree in business finance, I bought my first car. To my delight, my chronically disengaged father offered to take me car shopping so he could "show me how a car purchase is done." The impractical car I fell madly in love with was a used 1983 Toyota Celica. I bought it for about $3,200 in January 1988.

When we got the car home from the dealership, my dad took the time to show me all around my car, including popping the hood and explaining the engine parts and how the whole thing worked. I'm a gear-head so I was definitely interested, but I also just wanted to drive the dang thing. However, I'll never forget what my dad said to me, standing there in our dirt driveway, sporting his ridiculous Gilligan hat (my dad was a bit eccentric):

"Kid, most people drive around in their car with no idea how it works. Understanding the basics about how your car works will save you a lot of trouble and headaches. It will also help you have intelligent discussions with car mechanics and help you care for the vehicle so it runs well for a long time. There's a lot of miles left in this car, if you take good care of it."

I didn't know it at the time, but the man's speech had laid the foundation for the work I fell madly in love with about fifteen years later.

Understanding how my car worked did everything my dad said. I changed my own oil and brake fluid, replaced the fan belt, replaced spark plugs that had become un-sparky, changed flat tires roadside, and replaced the sticky thermostat that was making the engine overheat. When I did occasionally bring it to a garage for some work outside of my abilities, and they started doing mechanic-speak, I spoke their language—not fluently, but well enough to communicate. This helped me have meaningful dialogue and make smart decisions surrounding the care of my car. Dad was right.

Your physical body is simply the vehicle your spirit gets to ride around in. Your body is a tiny fence around a little part of a glorious and complete idea. If we see the body as a means by which the world is transformed, and not an end in itself, this guides our thinking and perception to one that serves us, BodyMindSpirit. And if your body isn't well-cared-for, it's more likely to "break down." This creates symptoms on the continuum from mild (frequent burping) to medium (type 2 diabetes) to drastic (cancer). We can substitute bodies for cars in my dad's driveway speech to arrive at a solid mantra for honoring our body:

"Most people ride around in their body having no idea how it works. Understanding the basics about how your body works will save you a lot of trouble and headaches. It will also help you have intelligent discussions with healthcare practitioners, and help you care for your body so it runs well for a long time. There's a lot of miles left in that body, if you take good care of it."

A sentiment that I hear over and over in my work is, *"I had no idea that habit X affected my body that way. I've always just followed the diet, tried the trick touted on social media, followed my doctor's 'orders,' without understanding how the body works. What you've just told me, in a way I can understand it, changes everything."* Education can be empowering. Thanks to my dad, I'm an empowered car owner. Now, as part of my passionate work in BodyMind-Spirit health, I help people become empowered body owners.

Our bodies are magnificent and resilient, and I fell head-over-heels in love with biochemistry and cell biology in grad school. The human body is complex beyond what we can possibly imagine. Even with all that we've learned over the hundreds of thousands of years that we've been knocking around on this planet—all that we've experienced, research and insight from the brightest minds, and vast and deep scientific studies of the human body—we still know shockingly little. Although we've learned a great deal in comparison to 2,000 years ago—or even 100 years ago—our understanding and wisdom in relation to our physiology is still in its infant stages. The body is a vessel of wisdom filled with truth, and we still have much to uncover.

As one example, DNA is the code of life, yet we currently only comprehend the significance of 3 percent of our DNA. Science previously labeled the remaining 97 percent "Junk DNA"—as if any part of the code-of-all-life-on-Earth would be junk. We need to develop humility about what we don't know, instead of wanting power over the body. Our current medical paradigm depends largely on surgery and medications to "fix" the body as if it is only made up of disparate parts, as if we are "all-knowing" and can force the body back into balance. In truth, our bodies are part of Mother Nature, and Mother Nature has a history of persevering.

The good news is that much of what serves the body is inarguable because it is dictated by evolution. In my work with clients and large groups over the years, I have focused on the eight main elements of building physical health: food, hydration/oxygenation, sleep, movement, digestion, weight, hormone balance, and immunity. I call this building Body Sass.

Body Sass° is balance, integration, and harmony in the body—being clinically well and feeling good in our body. Whether a client is looking to heal from dis-ease, lose weight, or optimize their health, some combination of these Body Sass elements will inform our focus. Consider this chapter an introductory handbook for getting under the hood of your physical self—a guide to basic body care via the four most easily accessible of these success elements: food, hydration/oxygenation, sleep, and movement.

Fabulous Food

Homo erectus began walking upright over two million years ago, with our present species homo sapiens distinguishing itself from its ancestors about 200,000 years ago. For most of our existence, food was something we ate only for survival. In the last 100 years or so, it's become something that we mass manufacture and consume for other reasons, largely social and emotional. We now create diets, count macros, restrict, overeat, and deeply analyze our food intake with scientific studies. We even have industrial food, which I'm pretty sure is an oxymoron. Various whole foods fall in and out of favor with science, which I find wryly amusing because whole foods (aka nature) have been around millions of years longer than the scientists.

Don't get me wrong, I'm an out-of-the-closet science geek, and I deeply appreciate many of the things that science has done for us. However, as with any field of study or entity, when factions become ego-driven, commercialized, and/or driven by profits, the truth may no longer be honored. It's disturbing, for instance, that we have suddenly decided that certain health-building whole foods like eggs and butter make us sick, while we promote synthetic foods, like Ensure and margarine, which actually *do* make us sick.

To say the culture we've created around food is confusing is an understatement of epic proportions. In order to support you in honoring your body, we're going to *simplify*. First, let's explore some foundational concepts about the body. This is the human physiological version of the driveway tour of a car engine with my dad, and it's key to understanding the significance of food choices.

We build our body with food, water, and oxygen. Our complex, powerful, mysterious, and self-healing body takes in the macronutrients carbohydrate, fat, and protein, along with a vast array of micronutrients—vitamins, minerals, and phytochemicals—and, using them, builds, maintains, and balances itself. That bears repeating: it builds, maintains, and balances itself, with no instruction from our conscious mind. It's a self-organizing system. The food we eat builds our body, every day, for better or worse. We're an ambulatory interconnected blob of 50 trillion cells, and every minute of our lives, roughly 300 million cells die and are replaced with brand-spanking-new ones. You might wonder why we give a hoot about any of this. Here's what's hoot-worthy: we replace a staggering 432 billion cells each day. This means that every day presents us with an amazing opportunity to rebuild our body with the powerful raw materials in nutrient-dense whole foods. We can incrementally create new health for ourselves, every minute of each day. That, dear reader, is empowering.

Prior to reading *Beating Cancer with Nutrition,* I thought, like most folks, that we were born, grew into a bigger body, and then simply kept that same ol' body for life. I thought we ate to fill our stomachs. Most of us, when eating, are eating to please our taste buds and fill our grumbly stomachs. In actuality, we're building our body with what we put into it, and our stomach is only a middleman. Now that I know better, I'm still all about food that tastes good, *and* I simultaneously focus on my fifty trillion cells that are replacing themselves and growing using the materials I provide to them via my food choices.

So the question is, do we want to build a chips, cookies, and fast-food body (the ticket to weight gain, dis-ease, fatigue, and general malaise) or do we want to build a vegetables, nuts, and eggs body (the ticket to weight loss, health, energy, and vibrant living)? My food philosophy is simple: eat yummy-tasting whole foods that provide the body with maximum nutrition. That's it. Twelve words. We could just "peace-out" here, but due to our general confusion around food, I'm going to dig in a bit deeper. In my practice, I work with people to collaboratively create an individual food lifestyle that fits into their everyday lives while providing them with flexibility, nutrients, and satisfaction. My intention on these pages is not to lay out specific food rules but to provide an instructive framework that can support you in building a healthy body.

Many people think that healthy food tastes gross, is expensive, and is a lot of work. The reality is that health-building food can taste off-the-charts amazing, and even if it can cost a bit more and require a bit more in the way of time and planning, it's ultimately worth it. With regards to the cost (a complaint even from folks who can afford good food), I'm going to be lovingly blunt: we can pay now at the market, or we can pay later with increased medical costs or a diminished quality of life. I work with some young people (late teens or early twenties) who are already living their pay-later, so I'm not necessarily referring to when we're eighty years old.

One of the most important health-builders we have access to is real, nutrient-dense food, so it's worth a look at your expenses to uncover ways to funnel a few more of your hard-earned dollars toward building your Body Sass. Our tour through personal responsibility, self-worth, and self-care in the last three chapters, along with our discussion about habits in Chapter 2, will support you in shifting your food choices more toward Food Sass.

"What on earth is 'Food Sass?'" you may be wondering. **Food Sass**® is food that nutritiously, deliciously contributes to creating vibrant health. Not fake, imposter food—edible, at best—that fools our senses and leaves us with less energy, more fat, and ultimately poor health. Food Sass is, well, sassy. Let's get clear on the definition of Food Sass.

Food Sass \füd sas\ noun: whole, organic, nutrient-dense foods that are as *close to their original state as possible. Taste amazing. Most typically found at farm stands or around the perimeter of the market. Contain a combination of clean protein, healthy fats, and complex carbohydrates. Provide loads of phytochemicals, vitamins, and minerals in their original state. Contribute to a plant-slant food lifestyle that is enjoyable and flexible with plenty of variety.*

Understanding which foods *do* serve our health helps us rule out a doughnut as a health-building choice. A doughnut is not whole nor close to any original state; nor does it have any clean protein, healthy fats, or complex carbs. From the point of view of our fifty trillion cells, the doughnut is anti-health. However, a snack of an organic apple smeared with organic nut butter falls well within the Food Sass guidelines. Each day in my work, I get to be a guide of and witness to mind-blowing health turnarounds; most of them are largely due to committed, mindful changes in food lifestyle, especially ones that embrace food as enjoyment *and* as medicine. The philosophy, principles, and biochemistry behind Food Sass have nothing to do with fads, trends, packaged diet meals, or processed foods that are packaged to sound like health food. They have everything to do with food that fuels, heals, and delights our physiology and senses.

Shortly, we'll explore the most important tenets in eating for health, focusing largely on what to seek out. But first, we need to understand that *the food that we avoid is as important as the food we seek out.* Contrary to popular belief, taking a daily multivitamin doesn't make up for a daily breakfast of Pop-Tarts. Most multivitamins are made with synthetic compounds that were created in a lab to mimic what's found in nature, often focusing on the "active compound" in a vitamin. We need vitamins in their natural state, with all of their compounds and co-factors intact—from food. Those synthetic daily multivitamins aren't even doing what we think they're doing in our body. And, even if it's a whole-food-based multivitamin that we've chosen, it's still not erasing the effects of anti-health foods.

Although eating Food Sass all the time would be great, that goal is also not real-world doable for most people. I encourage applying the famous

"80/20 rule" to food intake, with 80 percent or more of our intake as Food Sass, and up to 20 percent as what I not-so-lovingly refer to as fake food—those anti-health foods that we just discussed. This includes all of the white flour, potatoes, corn, and sugar that permeate the 80,000+ industrial foods that line our supermarket aisles. Fake food further includes industrial fats such as heavily processed vegetable oils (canola, corn, cottonseed, soybean, safflower, and peanut oil), chemical sweeteners, soda and energy drinks, most fast foods, and the majority of protein/energy bars.

Please don't make this yet another area to feel stress about. The purpose of telling you this information isn't to guide you to perfect eating; it's to clear up the cultural confusion surrounding what builds health and what doesn't, using basic tenets and short lists. Remember that our 80/20 rule means that sometimes we eat that doughnut, but we know it for what it is: a health barrier. If we choose to eat it as part of our 20 percent, we enjoy it, and then we focus on filling in our 80 percent with health-building foods. In order to move toward an 80/20 rule, it becomes important to understand what builds health and what doesn't.

We've briefly discussed what doesn't build health, so what kind of food *does* bring balance to the body? Keeping the definition of Food Sass in mind as our foundation, let's look at a simple outline and follow it up with some specific ways you can get started. We've covered the idea of eating as much whole and organic food as possible. What else is important?

EAT MOSTLY VEGETABLES

Vegetables are rich in health-building fiber, vitamins, minerals, enzymes, and thousands of phytochemicals. They also encourage a more alkaline state in the body, offsetting the heavy consumption of foods that create an acidic state in the body, such as meat, grains, and sugar. The dark-green, leafy veggies are especially "cape-worthy" (they are Food Sass superheroes). Our optimal health is best supported by getting seven to nine servings of veggies a day, with a serving being one-half cup. That's four and a half cups of veggies a day—many folks don't even eat one. (And no, French fries and ketchup don't count.) Raw veggies provide an added bonus of enzymes that help with digestion, so munch away on those raw carrots and broccoli. Overcooking vegetables can deplete their nutrient content, especially if they're cooked in water.

CHOOSE FATS WISELY

It's impossible to lose body fat and build healthy cells without eating dietary fat. Dietary fat does not make us fat *if* we consume healthy fats, in moderation. Healthy fats boost our metabolism, contribute to weight loss, and help us absorb fat-soluble vitamins A, D, E, and K. They promote a healthy brain (our brain is 60 percent fat); allow our cell membranes to function properly (read: create health); and reduce inflammation. That's the short list of benefits. However, not all fats are created equally.

I suggest avoiding health-eroding fats such as hydrogenated or partially hydrogenated fats (trans fats), canola oil, soy oil, vegetable oil, corn oil, peanut oil, margarine, and fake butter. Instead, seek out fats such as butter, eggs, coconut oil, olive oil, avocados and avocado oil, and raw nuts.

Consuming essential fatty acids (EFAs)—omega-3 fats and omega-6 fats—is also important. They're called essential because we can't make them ourselves, unlike the many important fats we can manufacture in our body using the molecules of the fats that we ingest. We can get EFAs from sardines, wild-caught salmon, mackerel, wild game, pasture-raised eggs, grass-fed beef, pumpkin seeds, chia seeds, flaxseeds, nuts, and dark leafy greens such as spinach and chard. These fats are anti-inflammatory, which is important as we're living in an age with high incidence of chronic inflammatory diseases like heart disease, cancer, diabetes, and more.

CONSUME ANIMAL PROTEIN IN MODERATION, AND FROM ANIMALS LIVING NATURALLY

Between paleo (meat-heavy) and vegan (excludes anything that comes from an animal or insect, including eggs or honey), there's a middle way. As omnivores, we've evolved over millions of years to function well with some animal food sources. However, we need *far* less animal protein (white, red, finned, or otherwise) than we generally assume. If we choose to eat animal protein, a few times a week is plenty. Eggs from pastured hens, however, can be consumed daily and are rich in nutrients.

Please note: I'm making an effort in our food discussion to minimize discussion of biochemistry as related to food, despite it being one of my favorite subjects to geek out on. Yet I must say this: the demonization of dietary cholesterol has been twisted and magnified to a point of veritable insanity. It's not based on recent science. Our bodies make whatever cholesterol is lacking in our food intake because cholesterol is a vital compound in our biochemistry. We need it to survive. Now, off the soapbox and back to animal protein.

If we're going to consume animal flesh—chicken, deer, fish, pork, cow, turkey, bison—it's important, for many reasons, to seek out animals that have lived as naturally as possible. This means that they ate what they evolved eating—for instance bugs, seeds, and grass for a chicken. It also means they live in an environment that is closest to their natural one—out in sunshine for our chicken friend. A cow standing in a barn for the brief years of her industrial life—with bars keeping her head in place, eating soymeal, being injected with hormones and antibiotics, and being milked by a machine—will experience poor health. This is why an industrially farmed cow lives four short years while her pastured sister lives a long, healthy average of fifteen years. Unhealthy, mistreated animals make nutritionally inferior milk, eggs, and meat. In the same way that we do, they build their body, for better or for worse, from their food and environment.

Animal protein from wild or consciously farmed animals not only carries a better energetic into our systems, but is far richer in nutrients such as omega-3 fats, and doesn't carry pesticides and stress chemicals from an animal living a stressful life. This is all aside from the ethical question of industrial farming, which I believe is an important one to consider.

FOCUS ON FIBER

Our digestive tract functions optimally with about forty-five grams of fiber intake per day. However, most people are topping out at around ten to fifteen grams daily. Fiber reduces the risk of heart disease; protects against colon cancer and diverticulitis; improves bowel function; helps us regulate our blood sugar, which protects against type 2 diabetes and heart disease; feeds all of the health-promoting bacteria that live in our GI tract; helps us lose weight; and helps us feel full longer after eating. High-fiber food categories are veggies, fruits, legumes, oatmeal, seeds, and nuts. Some of the top high-fiber foods are berries, avocado, Brussels sprouts, cauliflower, broccoli, legumes (beans), oatmeal, sweet potatoes, onions, and almonds.

When increasing fiber intake, it's best to do so gradually over a few weeks and to pay attention to your body's signals. If you feel bloated or gassy, you need to ramp up more slowly. Note that introducing more fiber into your food lifestyle also requires a higher water intake to balance it.

CHOOSE CARBS CAREFULLY

Carbohydrates come in an array of forms, with varying nutritional values. For our purposes here, there are two main types of carbs: empty carbs and smart carbs. The empty-carb category contains commercial grains (including corn, which is a grain, not a vegetable); sugars; and white rice and potatoes. Empty carbs trigger weight gain and contain little in the way of nutrients and fiber. Some common forms of empty carbs are bread, pasta, cereal, crackers, bagels, muffins, doughnuts, cookies, bakery products, pizza, candy, potato and corn chips, and boxed cereal.

"What about the whole-wheat version of those things?"

Don't fall for the whole-wheat scam. The average piece of white bread has 0.7 grams of fiber and the average piece of whole wheat bread has 2 to 4 grams of fiber, and it has a similarly pitiful nutrient profile. It's labeled as "whole wheat" because it contains some amount of whole-grain fiber, but this is often very little. Bread and all of the whole-grain versions of the foods listed above, in general, live on the 20 percent side of our 80/20 rule. If we're shooting for forty-five grams of fiber per day, two to four grams isn't much, especially compared to a nutrient-dense food such as an avocado, which boasts ten grams.

Smart carbs that live on the 80 percent side of our 80/20 rule include veggies, legumes, fruits (in moderation), quinoa, oatmeal, brown and wild rice, and sprouted grain breads like Food for Life's Ezekiel Bread. When eating for weight loss and blood-sugar health, it's best to consume starchy smart carbs in moderation, including root veggies, oatmeal, legumes, brown rice, and sprouted grain breads. For fruit, it's best to limit yourself to one serving of fruit per day, or at least follow a guideline of eating veggies and fruits in a two-to-one ratio. Fruits are similarly plentiful in nutrients like veggies, but eat them with the caveat that also they contain ample fructose. Fructose is a special form of sugar that seems to lend more directly to weight gain than other sugars. An apple a day still helps keep the doctor away, but after you eat it, move on to your veggies.

LIMIT DAIRY AND DRUGS

Unfortunately for all us cheese lovers, most research has shown cow dairy products to be inflammatory. They are especially hard on our thyroid gland (which is the master of our metabolism) and our digestive tract (which absorbs our nutrients). Contrary to mass-media marketing fueled by industrial dairy producers, the most absorbable forms of calcium come from dark leafy greens, not from milk moustaches. Simply limiting dairy can be a step toward a better health experience.

Although we're well-served to avoid drugs in general, culturally accepted drugs such as caffeine, alcohol, and nicotine inhibit health too. One to two cups of coffee a day isn't a deal breaker, especially if consumed before noon, and a glass of wine a few nights a week isn't going to send us over the edge either. However, when we're consistently relying on coffee for fake energy during the day and alcohol to fake-relax us at night, our physiology and biochemistry can become stressed and imbalanced. This physiological stress and imbalance can lead to weight gain, mental stress, high blood pressure, type 2 diabetes, inflammation, and impaired liver and brain function. Again, you don't have to abstain from caffeine and alcohol to be healthy, but less is definitely better.

EAT LOCAL

Leaning toward locally grown foods when shopping naturally helps us to eat more in season. Why is this important? Much of the produce we find in our supermarkets is ten to fourteen days old and has been shipped an average of 2,000 miles. The nutrients in plant foods have a short shelf life, gradually depleting post-harvest. For instance, we *can* eat an apple that was picked ten months ago (which is common), since apples take a relatively long time to decompose; but many of the apple's nutrients would have long since disappeared. Eating local—strawberries and cucumbers in the summer and root veggies in the winter—means there's a much shorter time between harvest and your mouth. This translates into more nutrients and better taste. You also add the benefit of supporting local farms—healthy for us and healthy for our food chain.

FORGET THE CALORIE MYTH

The caloric content of food is a concept that folks can become over-focused on, and calorie counting can be tedious and stressful. Instead of counting calories, eat calories that count. Cultivate an understanding about food and your body because, at the end of the day, your health and weight are less about the number of calories in food and more about the quality of the food that you eat. You see, the effect of calories in our biochemistry, which is what we care about, depends largely on the nutrient makeup of food itself. A bagel and an avocado each have roughly 230 calories. The bagel, due to its size and density, is equivalent to four slices of bread. Further, like most refined grain products, that bagel is comparable to a candy bar in our digestive system about twenty-five minutes after we eat it. This is because an empty carbohydrate food like a bagel or pasta is quickly broken down into the same simple sugars that comprise a candy snack. It has no nutrients, is a one-way ticket to weight gain, and we're practically guaranteed to be hungry an hour later because empty carbs are, well, empty. Meanwhile, the avocado boasts ten grams of fiber, copious health-building monounsaturated fats, as well as vitamins and minerals. The fats and fiber help us feel full longer and help us lose weight, while blasting our cells with nutrients. A bagel and an avocado contain the same number of calories, but create different impacts in the body. As the saying goes, not all calories are created equally.

That said, it's good to know the caloric content of fake food. It's instructive to understand, for example, that the Starbucks java chip Frappuccino coffee that we pick up each day has close to 500 calories. Knowing this, we realize that we're *drinking* one whole quarter of our daily calories and receiving no nutrients from that beverage; and, we're still likely to eat as much as we would without the Frappuccino. If we keep up our Frappuccino habit, we're adding 3,500 nonnutritive liquid calories a week to our intake, which is akin to eating a whole extra day-and-a-half of calories (most folks require 2,000 to 2,500 calories a day). The result of this habit is fewer health-building nutrients and more body fat. This is an example of how calorie information can be helpful in helping us make informed choices about fake food.

NAVIGATE FOOD MINDFULLY

Nature provides food for life on Earth, and we thrive on that food. However, there are some exceptions and fine print that I should touch on. There are natural foods which, in certain quantities, may create trouble for us. For instance, some folks are sensitive to nightshade veggies such as tomatoes, potatoes, eggplant, and peppers. Further, there is some research and clinical theory showing that plant lectins can make us sick, due to the quantities in which we eat them. Lectins are compounds in plants that protect them from predators. Let's face it, to a plant, we're simply a big bug on two legs—plants would rather survive and reproduce than become our next meal. They produce lectins in amounts that are hazardous for bugs, and may be hazardous for us if we eat an abundance of high-lectin foods such as grains, legumes, tomatoes, and peppers.

Additionally, some people become intolerant of, or sensitive to, foods when they have a compromised intestinal lining. Eating these foods then results in them having symptoms, which are typically dose-dependent. This means that symptoms are in proportion to the amount of the offending food eaten. These sensitivities are different from food allergies, where any amount of the food causes severe, life-threatening reactions in the body. A simple way to find out if you have issues with nightshades or lectins, or intolerances to other foods, is to remove the group you suspect may be creating symptoms for a week and notice how you feel. Then, notice how you feel when you add the group back in.

In addition to understanding the food choices that build or erode health, it's also helpful to mindfully incorporate some healthy eating tactics. For instance, people often balk at the idea of pizza living on the 20 percent side of the 80/20 equation. I know; pizza is yummy. I explain to them that it doesn't mean we never eat pizza; it means that we do it craftily. If we have a big salad or a veggie side dish with our pizza—and we eat the veggies first—we can still get our beloved pizza but we'd fill up on the health-building items first. We still honor our pizza desire, but we hopefully end up eating only one or two slices instead of seven. In general, I suggest eating the healthiest things on your plate first and saving the 20 percent items for last.

Portions of meat and starches are best kept to the size of our palm or smaller, while portions of veggies can be as big as we choose. Then, we eat until we're satisfied (about 75 percent full), not stuffed. We need to eat slowly to allow time for our stomach to tell our brain that it's satisfied. Please know that it's okay to not be a member of the clean-plate club. If your hunger has abated, stop eating. Several small meals over the course of our day will help right-size and nourish our body more than a few big meals.

Finally, when we feel pulled to emotional eating, we give ourselves the gift of time. Allow a space between the impulse and the action, and drink two cups of water in that space. Then, do something healthy that makes you feel good, like taking a short walk, reading, breathing a few deep breaths of fresh air, or organizing your sock drawer (if organizing makes you feel satisfied). Doing this repeatedly can rewire the reward center of our brain, significantly reducing emotional eating.

No set diet could be entirely correct for all people. I invite you to explore the boundaries suggested in this chapter and uncover what supports you in feeling your best. Expanding your palate, prioritizing healthy food, and eating for health is something you'll get better at over time, and it's the rock-solid foundation of a healthy BodyMindSpirit. To get started, pick one or two areas of focus, reread Chapter 2 on habit formation, and go slow and steady.

Please, remember to be gentle and flexible with yourself. Enjoying food—the food itself and the socialization that often accompanies food—is part of our relationship with food, and there's certainly no need to change that.

O_2 and H_2O

Food is one thing we build our body with, and water (H_2O) and oxygen (O_2) are the other two. Unlike food, with its layers of taste and nutrition, water and oxygen are one-size-fits-all. They're also deal breakers, in the sense that we die if we go without them for even a short time. We can live without food for up to forty days. However, we can only live without water for two to seven days, and we die within ten minutes or so without oxygen. Given that we can't live without them, if you're reading this, then you're getting enough oxygen and water to sustain life. However, even if you're not one of the 844 million people worldwide who don't have access to clean, safe drinking water, the estimates are that 75 percent of Americans (90 percent of whom *do* have access to clean, safe drinking water) are still chronically dehydrated.

Moreover, even though oxygen is a breath away, thanks to our plankton and plant friends, many of us don't breathe in a way to optimize our oxygen intake. Let's take a closer look at oxygen and water.

O_2: OXYGEN

When we're babies, we breathe naturally. We breathe in and out deeply, with the ribs and belly going in and out to accommodate the deep pull and release on the diaphragm. You see, our lungs don't actually *do* the breathing, as they have no muscles. Instead, our lungs get breathed by our diaphragm, the big, dome-shaped muscle that separates our chest cavity (where our lungs and heart live) from our abdomen (where our digestive and reproductive organs live).

Two things happen as babies grow into adults. (Well, in truth a lot of things happen, but we're focusing on the two that relate to breathing.) One, we become socialized to hold in our stomach to enhance the appearance of svelteness. Two, many of us experience chronic stress, which can lead to shallow breathing. When we breathe this way, we only fill and empty just the tippy-top of the lungs. These two things, along with our increasingly stationary existence, lead to less-than-optimal oxygenation of our bodies.

We can get by with less-than-optimal intake of oxygen, as with many of the other contributors to our health, but we're likely setting ourselves up for trouble many years out. Shallow breathing lowers white blood cell count (immunity), increases likelihood of panic attacks, aggravates respiratory problems, and is a precursor for cardiovascular issues. Cancer cells prefer an anaerobic environment, which is biochemistry-talk for "cancer cells don't like oxygen." Increasing our oxygen content makes our body a more hostile environment for growing cancer cells; and it makes any cancer cells we already have sad and feeble, making us healthier. Finally, shallow breathing (using chest instead of belly) over-uses the muscles in our chest, neck, and shoulders, which can translate into neck pain, headaches, and being more injury-prone.

On the flip side, diaphragmatic breathing (recruiting our bellies and ribs instead of our chest muscles) has been shown to lower blood pressure, reduce our heart rate, increase our energy, relax our muscles, and inhibit the stress response. Recreating the habit of natural diaphragmatic breathing is a free and easy way to support good health.

H_2O: WATER

It's well known that our bodies are 60 to 80 percent water; the common adage is that we need to drink eight cups (64 oz.) of water a day. I'm not sure where that number came from, but it falls short of our physiological needs. We excrete ten to fifteen cups (80 to 120 oz.) of water a day while living a relatively sedentary life, and much more when we're engaged in movement and exercise. We lose body water via urine, feces, perspiration, and breathing. In fact, we excrete four to eight cups of water (32 to 64 oz.) *just by breathing* during an average sedentary day, and much more when exercising. When we then add the diuretic effects of alcohol and caffeine, our poor little cells are absolutely parched.

Research suggests that 75 percent of Americans are chronically dehydrated. I've had clients with digestive dysfunction, muscle cramping, headaches, or fatigue who simply increased their water intake and healed their malaise. Game. Changer. I'm not going to list all the things that water does to support our health. I imagine that you can appreciate that if we're made of 60 to 80 percent water, it's involved in pretty much everything in our bodies. The one specific bit of information I will share is that toxins leave our body largely via water. If we're chronically dehydrated, this limits the buses (water) that the toxins can ride out on, causing our toxin-removal system to get clogged like a one-exit parking lot after a country music concert in Nashville. Dehydration creates a toxic burden in the body, encouraging inflammation, lowered immunity, and disease.

My work in guiding BodyMindSpirit health and joy, as well as my personal experience, has proven that it's not enough to simply say, *"Wow, I need to drink more water. I'll get on that."* The question is *"What new habits and routines do I need to create to support my desire to be optimally hydrated?"* Personally, I'm not an on-task water drinker by nature. This means I needed to create intentional habits around hydration. I drink three cups (with lemon, for healthy bile function) when I get up; I typically have six cups of herbal tea by 1:00 pm; and I have a glass container that holds three cups of water that I drink in the afternoon. These habits add up to about twelve cups of water a day. I don't typically drink water with my meals because I don't want to dilute my digestive juices. I don't drink much after dinner because I want to limit my nighttime bathroom visits. Another factor to figure in to your hydration habits is that some liquids are dehydrators, such as caffeine and alcohol. You'll need even more water if you drink caffeinated and/or alcoholic beverages.

Finally, we could delve into deep detail about the types of water you could drink. Let's keep it simple: the worst is tap water and the best is mineral or purified water. The best intersection of healthy and inexpensive is filtered tap water. Most tap water contains chlorine and fluoride, which have been linked to health issues, including cancer and brain damage. Filtering via reverse osmosis or deionizers can remove some of tap water's impurities like these chemicals. Remember, as with any of these changes, you can start small. Any kind of water is better than chronic dehydration. Adequate water is essential for health, as is adequate sleep.

Sleep Your Way to Success

Creating habits to support adequate amounts of restful sleep at night is foundational to our health. Sleep is important: when we feel rested, we're productive and more able to positively engage with our day and the people in it. Sleep is also important for many, much deeper health reasons, including strengthening immunity, clearing and regulating emotions, digestive-system maintenance, brain-cell creation, weight loss, healthy gene expression, and avoiding or healing depression. What I've come to understand about sleep is that our BodyMindSpirit requires downtime to reset, recalibrate, and rest in order to run interference against sickness and disease. We think we're lying down at night only because we're tired, but sleep is something that we need at our most fundamental level to create optimal health and joy.

The good news is that most folks understand that sleep is important because we feel lousy when we don't get enough of it, or get poor quality sleep. Most current research shows that if we're getting any less than seven and a half hours of quality sleep per night, then we're sleep deficient.

If you find yourself struggling with sleep, here are some tips to help you improve this essential aspect of your well-being:

RELAX BEFORE BEDTIME

Try to avoid stimulating activities at night; instead, dim your lights and calm yourself in the hour or two before bedtime. It can help to have a relaxing bath, listen to quiet music, or read. For most of us, it's best not to watch scary, disturbing, or violent television—including news programming—in the few hours before bed. We may also want to avoid starting a new project at the end of the day or getting involved in an emotional situation (an argument, for example), if we can avoid it.

SET A SCHEDULE

Our sleep/wake cycle, which is controlled by the hypothalamus gland in our brain, is part of our circadian rhythm; it's guided by the rising and setting of the sun. Although it may not be possible to follow nature's rhythms as we did prior to electricity, it's still best to go to bed at a set time each night and get up at roughly the same time each morning. On days off from work, it's best not to sleep in more than one or two hours later than we do on a workday, or we'll disrupt our sleep cycle. If your sleep schedule has been disrupted (such as with jet lag), you can try one to two grams of melatonin before bed for a few nights to help your brain reset.

AVOID CAFFEINE, NICOTINE, AND ALCOHOL

Caffeine, chocolate, colas, and cigarettes can stimulate our brain and prevent it from recognizing when it's time to sleep. It's best if we avoid the caffeine in coffee, tea, chocolate, and soda after 12:00 pm. Alcohol, a depressant, may send us off to sleep more quickly, but it's likely to interrupt our sleep cycle in the middle of the night because it dehydrates us and disrupts our blood sugar.

CONTROL YOUR SLEEP ENVIRONMENT

Maintain a comfortable temperature, preferably around 65°F/18°C or cooler, and perhaps crack a window wherever you sleep. Body temperature drops at night, so keep your feet warm with a hot water bottle, or wear socks in bed (quite sexy). Keep your bedroom dark, uncluttered, and soothing. Wear comfortable 100 percent natural-fiber nightclothes that allow your body to better regulate its temperature. Be sure to have a comfortable, supportive mattress and a comfortable pillow that doesn't crick your neck or spine. Block out noises and angle the face of your alarm clock so you can't see it. It doesn't help you feel relaxed and sleepy to look at the clock at night when you can't sleep.

MOVE IT, BABY

To help yourself be ready to sleep, try to have at least twenty to thirty minutes of physical activity daily, especially during the early part of the day. Compared to sedentary folks, people who exercise not only sleep longer and more deeply, but also fall asleep much faster. Resistance training, cardiovascular exercise, walking, yoga, and functional stretching exercises can all help to improve sleep efficiency and quality. We'll discuss movement in more detail shortly.

EAT HEALTH-BUILDING FOODS

We're back to the importance of Food Sass. Fake Food can disrupt sleep, and sugar in particular is a notorious sleep disruptor. Folks who engage in my various clean-eating programs are blown away by the restful sleep that accompanies this kind of food lifestyle. Avoid overeating in the evening, and finish eating at least two hours before bedtime to avoid weight gain and promote sound sleep.

REDUCE YOUR LEVELS OF CHRONIC STRESS

Stress is a top disruptor of our sleep patterns. This may sound depressing since we often feel as if our lives are stressful. I have great news: it's possible to re-educate your nervous system so to better respond to stress. Meditation, frequent deep breathing exercises, mindfulness, and stress resilience are some of the ways you can reduce stress and improve sleep. Stay tuned for more on this in the next chapter.

EXPERIMENT WITH PROFESSIONAL INTERVENTIONS

Massage therapy, acupuncture, chiropractic manipulation, osteopathy, and many other physical therapies—sometimes covered or partially covered by health insurance—can be effective treatments for insomnia. If you're feeling depleted, you need a good holistic approach to filling your cup. You could experiment with a combination of some of the above strategies to replete yourself. If you're depressed or anxious, you may benefit from psychological counseling.

I invite you to put in the time and care to create habits and lifestyle choices that support restful, health-building sleep. Our sleep quality changes because of many factors—food, stress, hydration, anxiety, weight, hormones, exercise, breathing, and others—making it important that we adapt as needed in order to maintain our sleep sweet spot.

Joyful Movement

You may have noticed that this section isn't called "exercise." I prefer the word *movement* over the word *exercise* because, for most people, exercise conjures images of intimidating weight rooms, boring cardio equipment, and doing something out of a sense of grim obligation. *"I'm going to go put in time on the treadmill"* or *"I'm heading out to slog through my run"* and *"No pain, no gain."* Oh boy, sign me up for all of that (sarcasm intended). The word *movement*, for many folks, seems to allow more room for fun. As such, I suggest you say goodbye to your exercise workout and say hello to finding *movement you love.*

Movement is essential for the entirety of our being, BodyMindSpirit. I read something in a biology book once that will forever ring in my head: *"Each day, we are instructing our body to either build up or break down, via our choice to be sedentary or active."* When we're active, we tell our fifty trillion cells that we need to stay strong and healthy. When we're sedentary, we tell our body, *"My needs for you are dwindling."* Yikes.

Consider our first 200,000 years on this planet—you know, the whole hunter, gatherer, and manual labor mojo. We needed to move to stay alive. Movement boosts our metabolism, burns fat, builds muscle, reduces the negative effects of stress, strengthens our cardiovascular system, moves our lymph system (which is key in our immunity), improves sleep, and—by creating a more oxygenated environment in the body—discourages cancer cells. And that's the short list.

Movement, like all things, runs along a continuum of effectiveness from a health standpoint. Although I'm not a trained exercise expert, I know enough through my lifelong experiences as a committed movement veteran, research, and my collaboration with trained exercise experts, to feel confident offering you sound basics, which is all most of us need. There are five main aspects that a comprehensive movement habit will include:

1. Cardio

2. Resistance

3. Recruiting

4. Flexibility

5. Approach

Let's look at how you can develop your *Movement I Love* lifestyle in a way that incorporates all five of those core aspects.

1. Cardio: *Get your heart rate and breathing amped up.*

Take some time and care when finding out what kind of cardio movement you love (or at least like) doing. I have friends and clients who are in love with spin class, rock climbing, hiking, mixed martial arts, intentional walking, cycling, yoga, ultimate Frisbee, rebounding (mini-trampoline), dancing, and swimming. That's not an exhaustive list, so I encourage you to explore, be creative, and to find out what you love. Then do that thing, or those things, consistently.

You might also try high-intensity interval training, or HIIT, a short ten- to twenty-five-minute cardio workout with many variations; some research is saying it's more effective and better for us than the classic long-form cardio.

2. Resistance: *Lift heavy stuff.*

Weight-bearing movement, also known as resistance training, is important for keeping us strong for everyday life, as well as for accelerating fat loss, increasing metabolism, and increasing bone density. Options for resistance training include free-weight routines, sandbag training, resistance bands, kettlebell and medicine ball training, and gymnastics-based bodyweight training. Any of these allows for effective, whole-body, functional strength movement in twenty minutes or less.

Ideas for how to create safe movement with any of these modes of resistance training can easily be found online, or through consult with a personal trainer. If you're new to resistance training, it's best to get professional guidance. It's fairly easy to hurt ourselves if we have poor form when lifting heavy things. Many of us who have lifted a heavy object off the ground by using only our back, instead of involving our legs, have learned this the hard way.

3. Recruiting: *Activate the full range of muscle fibers.*

When doing resistance training, focus on bringing your body through its full range of motion—the full movement potential of your joints. More muscle fibers are recruited and activated on an as-needed basis as we move through our full range of motion, while using the heaviest weight with which we can complete eight repetitions, while maintaining safe and proper form.

Muscle-recruitment philosophy can also be brought into cardio training by intentionally bringing your body through the full range of motion required by whatever activity you've chosen. For instance, I can walk by sluffing my feet along. Or I can walk by intentionally creating long strides, holding my core abdomen muscles firm, my chest forward and up (imagine a string attached to your sternum gently pulling up and allow your shoulders to relax back and down), and mindfully flexing my quads (thigh muscles) and glutes (butt muscles). The nonsluffing version is recruiting more muscle fibers.

4. Flexibility: *Encourage muscle suppleness and joint mobility.*

Flexibility training—static stretching, functional stretching, yoga, and Pilates are some forms of this—is key to the first three core aspects. Not only does flexibility help us move more easily and comfortably through our daily lives; it enhances our ability to do our best cardio, resistance training, and recruitment of muscle fibers—and it helps us do all that with fewer injuries. That's right, science has shown that the incidence of injury decreases when we include regular flexibility training in our movement habits due to our enhanced ability to move unimpeded through a wider range of movement.

5. Approach: *It's all in your mind.*

Your mind has two important jobs in relation to movement. One, as in the walking example, is that it keeps movement mindful, for maximum effect. Movement is more beneficial to the body and mind when we remain focused on *intentional* movement. Among other things, when we focus our mind on the muscles that we're using during movement, our muscles perform better.

Two, once you've invested the time to set yourself up for happy movement, decide how many days you are committing to engage in intentional movement; ideally you'll work up to four to six days per week. Then, each day, wake up and ask yourself which of your movement choices you'll engage with that can work with your schedule. *"Which movement would make me happiest today?"*

That's it. No schedules, long-term planning, performance tracking, self-flagellation, willpower, or military discipline required. Simply you and what you're in the mood for. This is how fitness becomes joyful self-care, instead of something that you hold over your head, drag yourself through, and eventually quit. It's a reframe from *go exercise* (heavy sigh) to *go have fun* or *go have some me-time* or *go decompress*. Much happier.

Finally, one more important aspect of movement is simply decreasing how much we sit. Americans sit an average of thirteen hours a day. When we add the eight hours of sleeping we should get, that means we can be sedentary for twenty-one of our twenty-four hours. From an evolutionary standpoint, it was a hot minute ago that we spent our days in almost constant movement, which means that our biology hasn't adjusted to our abruptly introduced stationary lifestyle. In my work with corporations and their employees, we talk about standing or moving for at least ten minutes out of each hour. I recommend trying to conduct walking meetings, getting a standing desk, or running up and down the stairs a few times during a work break.

Our body is built for movement and it yearns for movement, so find creative ways to move throughout your day. Think of movement as a way to restore energy, willpower, and metabolism, while promoting restful sleep. Oh yes, and it helps in weight management too. I invite you to spend the time and care to create a movement philosophy, and menu of activities, that you're happy with. This will change your relationship with movement and serve your health and joy, BodyMindSpirit, for life.

Honor Your Body

In my functional and integrative work with people who have health issues, my question is this: *"Why is the body doing that?"* This is a very different question from, *"How can we stop that from happening?"* Understanding the difference between these two questions has the power to completely change the way we approach our health journey. Allow me to explain.

A few decades back, I went to a gastroenterologist—a medical doctor who specializes in digestive dysfunction—to try to get to the bottom of why I had been suffering with intermittent digestive issues for the past fifteen years. I never knew when the bloating, discomfort, long and painful visits to the bathroom, and exhaustion was going to hit. During my eight minutes with the doc, he asked me about my symptoms and wanted to test for lactose intolerance (which came back negative) and to perform an exploratory colonoscopy. When I came back for my next appointment, post-colonoscopy, the doctor spent eleven minutes with me, during which he told me that I "had IBS-C" and handed me three prescriptions for medications that would control the episodes. The question he was asking was, *"How can we stop these symptoms from happening?"*

Please first know that the point of this discussion is not to pick on doctors, who are mostly beholden to a system ruled by the pharmaceutical and health-insurance industries, but instead to share with you a different philosophy of approaching dysfunction in the body. America's increased rate of chronic disease and tandem skyrocketing health-insurance costs are pleading for a new philosophy and approach; that's the focus of our discussion here. There are several things wrong with the typical medical interaction described in the last paragraph. First, open-minded curiosity is the surest path to insight and wisdom. This means that in order to gather data, we must ask good questions; a good place to start is the umbrella question, *"Why is the body doing that?"* The thing is, our bodies are so intelligent and adaptive that an organ can become as much as 60 percent dysfunctional before we experience noticeable symptoms.

This astounding adaptability means, for instance, that my liver—the largest internal organ that's involved in over 500 metabolic processes in the body, and is known in Chinese medicine as The Commanding General of the Body—could be doing only 41 percent of its job, and I may have no related symptoms. This is masterful. Can you imagine if the driver of an eighteen-wheeler was only doing 41 percent of her job while rocketing forty tons of machinery and cargo among thousands of passenger vehicles on the highway? I cringe to think of the death and disaster that would ensue. However, this eighteen-wheeler example is not synonymous with the wise and adaptable body.

Our body's complex integration creates compensations to offset things that aren't working right. In our body's constant striving for healing and balance—for the most optimal homeodynamic state possible in any given moment—it will rob Peter to pay Paul as needed. Over time, though, this starts to cause far-reaching problems, and that's when we get symptoms.

Symptoms are messengers that communicate from body to mind, allowing our mind to register that there's a problem and go to work—via actions from us—bringing balance back to our BodyMindSpirit system. A symptom is a message. Unfortunately, we often shoot the messenger. Moreover, I'll go out on a limb here and share that many of the modern dysfunctions that we call diseases are, in fact, symptoms. Type 2 diabetes, heart disease, IBS, fibromyalgia, migraines, dental cavities—these are big symptoms trying to bring us a message about dysfunction in the body. For instance, type 2 diabetes is a disease-name that we've attached to the symptom of insulin resistance. It shows up as chronically elevated blood sugar on blood tests. But these results or symptoms don't mean that we're diseased; instead, they indicate that we need to change the environment in the body to invite balance. In the case of type 2 diabetes, this most often means reducing our intake of empty carbs via a Food Sass 80/20 lifestyle, and engaging in daily movement.

Our focus, medically and culturally, is often on getting rid of the symptom, when that symptom is an important message that needs to be decoded. Certain groups of symptoms often cluster around dysfunction in a specific organ or system of the body; taking careful stock of symptom clusters can sometimes be helpful in pointing us in the right direction. Our job is not to suppress symptoms or attack illness but to decode symptoms and then get busy stimulating and supporting the natural forces of healing.

For instance, if we get frequent headaches, we typically take painkillers, such as ibuprofen. Instead of repeatedly squashing the messenger, an instructive question would be, *"Why am I getting so many darn headaches?"* We might investigate hydration, hormones, food intolerances, seasonal allergies, sleep deprivation, and a myriad of other things, including a brain scan. For example, when my stepdaughter Carolyn was a young college student, I worked with her as she bravely investigated food sensitivities and found relief from her symptom cluster of chronic migraines, stomach issues, and sinus issues. Scores of clients have had similar experiences over the years. Taking ibuprofen for chronic headaches is similar to continually wearing earplugs in a car so as not to hear the loud rattling noise coming from its engine. A better approach would be to ask good questions about engine function and find out what's causing that noise. Because while we're wearing those earplugs, the problem is likely only getting worse.

This all requires time, of course. Synthesizing comprehensive data—such as lab-test results, symptoms and their clusters, and background health history—and then combining it with a deep knowledge of how a BodyMind-Spirit organism works takes time—a lot more time than eight minutes, which is often how long the average medical appointment lasts.

Circling back to my IBS story, given that food builds our body, food choices are a key question when we're not well. This is *especially* true for digestive issues, because not only do we build the cells of that system with food but, unlike, say, our respiratory system or our brain, our food also directly touches our digestive tract.

Although I had yet to embark on my formal training in biochemistry and pathophysiology back then, I was far enough into my passion and research in health to find it particularly disturbing that my gastroenterologist didn't ask me a single question about my food lifestyle. Further, IBS isn't a disease. It's a constellation of symptoms that has been given a medical label so that a special code (an IDC code) can be attached to it that indicates which medications can be prescribed. Of this, I was aware; and despite still being green behind the ears, I wasn't resonating with the doctor's approach and declined the medications. I didn't want to merely stop my symptoms—while also upsetting other balances in my body with chemicals—I wanted to heal. The abbreviated version of the story is that I stopped eating soy and gluten, and the "IBS disease" disappeared overnight, after fifteen years of suffering, and never came back.

Personally and professionally, I've been party to hundreds of these scenarios where foundational healing is bypassed in favor of the quick-and-easy fix of silencing symptoms. Instead of going after these silver-bullet approaches, we need to ask: what is the body trying to tell us? What has been disrupted in the environment of the body or mind that has led to dysregulation? These are the questions that honor the body and invite healing. They move us away from suffering and toward health and joy. Your body is a hard-working and loyal vehicle, majestic and mysterious in every way possible—and wired for healing. I invite you to invest in it.

Remember: small things are big things. You might ask yourself which habits that we've discussed in this chapter you might start for your desired evolution toward better health. Maybe you can shift your environment to better support those habits. As always, personal responsibility, self-worth, and self-care are the pillars that support our evolution toward the most healthy, joyful version of ourselves. In the end, the actual information around honoring our body isn't terribly complicated; it's that the change in regards to how we act with food, water, breathing, sleep, and movement can seem hard. Creating change has to do with our mind and our habits. In the next two chapters, we'll delve into mind and spirit, as we expand our sense of self beyond our masterful body—for the sake of our well-being as well as that of the world around us. A more deep and juicy exploration of mind is exactly where we're headed.

CHAPTER 7:

TEND YOUR MIND

"If the mind is happy, not only the body but the whole world will be happy. So one must find out how to become happy oneself. Wanting to reform the world without discovering one's true self is like trying to cover the whole world with leather to avoid the pain of walking on stones and thorns. It is much simpler to wear shoes."

—SRI RAMANA MAHARSHI

Our entire life experience is filtered through the miraculous, powerful, and mysterious part of ourselves that we call *mind*. Our mind is the central hub of our life experience, and it functions as either bridge or barrier, depending on how we use it, moment to moment. Are we using our mind in a flexible and coherent way, encouraging integration of experience? Or are we leaning toward the extremes of either chaos or rigidity in the mind, creating suffering? Harnessing the power of the mind is where everything starts, where it ends, and where everything in between gets processed.

In order to live consciously, joyfully, and creatively as the complex work of art that we are, we need to have some understanding of the raw mental material we have to work with. In order to create our life experience—our moment-to-moment personal reality—with intention, we must become interested in, and attentive to, the manner in which we use our mind. Otherwise, our life experience will seem to just haphazardly happen to us.

For instance, we just spent an entire chapter exploring how to create and maintain health and balance in the body—a worthwhile discussion. However, all that has the potential to create health or dis-ease in the body—all of the choices we make, all of our habits, all of our self-talk about those choices and habits, and all of our intentions—are within the realm of mind.

Most diets discuss what to eat and why, without addressing what's happening in the mind. This is why 97 percent of diets fail within two years. When I guide people toward healing, better health, weight loss, and joy, the mind is a central discussion. We talk about changing one's relationship with food and self-care. We move from mind as barrier toward mind as bridge. We work with the powerful healing forces of the human organism—body, mind, and spirit working together. In the final analysis, in most cases, it's not primarily the body, but the mind that's in need of healing.

We started this book talking about mind in Chapter 2, and learning to tend the mind is threaded throughout this book. This chapter on mind is logistically central in Part Two and central in the book because it's central to health, joy, and personal evolution. And the best place to start a more in-depth inquiry on mind is to attempt to define the mind.

As with the glorious body, we're still on the very tippy-edge of understanding our mind—what it is, where it is, how it works, and how it affects and interacts with our other aspects of body and spirit. The tricky part is, what can we learn about mind, using our minds? That's a mind bender, indeed. I will not be handing over some neatly boxed, wrapped, and ribbon-tied package of a definition. There are people who have spent, and are spending, their entire life working to make inroads into our knowledge of the nature of mind. Rather, I will share what I've come to understand about mind via personal and professional inquiry and through study and research.

Meet Your Mind

Many folks think of the concepts of mind and brain as interchangeable. We fleshed that out a bit earlier, and it's time to reengage in that inquiry, with a bit of repetition to assist with understanding this complex topic. Our brain is a highly complex organ that sits inside the protective shelter of our skull, bobbling around at the top of our body. The human brain is the most complex physical object that we've uncovered in our solar system to date. Our brain, like the rest of our body, is built with food, oxygen, and water. It's made of about 60 percent fat and is fed by thousands of miles of blood vessels, sucking up around 20 percent of all the energy our body creates. The brain is partly akin to a computer that runs our body, all day every day, working to keep our hormones balanced, regulating fight-or-flight response, releasing neurotransmitters, pulling our hand away when it touches a hot surface, regulating breathing and heartbeat, and gazillions of other things. It also houses areas that science has associated with various thinking functions, such as perception, motor control, motivation, learning, and memory. It's a compilation of eighty-six billion interconnected neurons and synapses, along with other cell types, that interact with our entire body and with our complex and ever-changing environment.

Powerful stuff.

While the brain lives in our skull, whatever mind is, it's definitely *not* limited to the physical space between our ears. I suspect that it's whole-body at the very least. Much more probable is that mind also exists between beings and in relation to something a lot bigger than us. Meaning, the mind may not be only within us, it's likely between us and around us as well. I'm not suggesting that brain and mind are unrelated, but instead that they are different yet deeply interdependent aspects of our human experience. As we move into defining mind, an easy way to grasp this concept of brain/mind is by reviewing the basics of how a television or TV works.

A TV is a sophisticated electronic device made of visible working parts, and the brain is a sophisticated organ made of visible working parts. The electronic information that flows through the TV and into your auditory and visual senses brings the TV alive. In a similar way, the flow that we call mind is received by the brain and our entire being, bringing life and meaning to our existence. A working definition of mind, with the ground-breaking work of psychiatrist Daniel J. Siegel, PhD, at its core, could be: *Mind is all that relates to our subjective felt experience of being alive, to our thoughts and feelings, and to our consciousness. It's a self-organizing and emergent property of interconnected information and Energy flow happening within our entire brain and body, between humans, and with the entire natural world in which we live. We can experience the mind and we can direct it, but we can't always control it.* Stunning.

There's a lot to chew in that big mouthful. First, let's unpack the word *consciousness* a bit, which is an important concept in our exploration. I say *a bit* because consciousness, as we'll use it in this context, is widely recognized as one of the biggest mysteries of life. How is it that a seamless and never-ending array of sensations, thoughts, thinking, emotions, memories, intuitions, and knowings arise in us? How is it that we're aware that we're aware? Beats the heck out of me, so let's use a definition that summarizes what science and wisdom traditions have uncovered thus far, while knowing that this definition is in its infancy. **Consciousness** can be loosely thought of as our recognized mind functions, such as our five senses, thought function, emotional processing, and memory; plus intuition, insight, and our increasing awareness of the flabbergasting mystery of everything around us and within us. It's all this plus our being aware that we're aware of all that. Amazing. And we've just gotten started.

Immediately following the mention of consciousness in our Siegel-inspired definition of mind is the idea of a "self-organizing and emergent property." Self-organization emerges in complex systems when the whole has properties that its parts don't have. Mathematical theory describes the process of self-organization as the way a complex system regulates its own becoming. We can create bridges (facilitate) or barriers (impede) to self-organized systems, but self-organization is a natural process that arises from complex systems such as mind as they flow and shift. A good mental picture that helps us understand this is the way in which water flows down a tub drain. Instead of all bunching up or randomly rushing down, it organizes into a swirl of water that exits the tub in an organized fashion. It self-organizes. We can create a barrier by sticking a finger into that swirl and mess up the orderly exit of the water, but when we take our finger out, it self-organizes again.

Next, let's get clear on "interconnected information and Energy flow." The "e" in Energy is capitalized to differentiate it from the energy we've discussed up to this point. This is different from the energy we have when we wake up from a nap; or that is created from food, oxygen, and water to drive our muscles and metabolism; or that we get from a double espresso. This **Energy-with-a-capital-E** is the very stuff that creates all that surrounds us—the organizing Energy of the universe. Everything is created from this Energy; it can be neither created nor destroyed, and it forms and instructs everything from thoughts to stones to beetles to radio waves to plankton to human tissue. Information and Energy are tightly connected. Brain, mind, and relationships are three aspects of one reality, which is the flow of information and Energy.

I call this a working definition because, although it includes the most recent research and discoveries into mind, we're still in our infantile stages of understanding mind. The aspects of mind have been sliced and diced by various studies, experts, and groups in interesting ways. As one example, the mind activity that helps me figure out how to best pack the trunk of my car for a trip, and the mind activity that led Mozart to create his first complex musical compositions at age four—do these come from the same place? They're both information and Energy flow, but they feel like quite different things. The realm of mind begets more questions than answers; but all complexity aside, our integrated mind—and the engaged and intentional use of thought—is the most powerful tool available to us. Thoughts are powerful directors of Energy and, as such, they often manifest as crystallized, more dense Energy, such as events and physical things.

Our mind is our greatest tool and bridge, yes, and it can also be our greatest enemy and barrier when we use it to keep ourselves in suffering, which we all do to varying degrees. One important facet of this barrier aspect of mind is our **messy personhood** which, to be clear, is a term I made up. Psychologists, philosophers, and others who concern themselves with the study of mind often use the term *ego* to discuss the part of the mind that is responsible for our sense of being a separate personal identity who uniquely strives and suffers. Over the years, I've found that the term *ego* can get confusing for folks as they equate it with "egotistical," as in, "Holy moly, does he have a big ego." The term *messy personhood,* with the word *messy* being infused with love and acceptance, feels less confusing and more accurate. Persons aren't messy in their essence; we're not born messy. The messy part happens in our minds. We feel separate from everything around us and therefore feel the need to protect what's "ours." Because we're deeply interconnected with all of the beings and life around us, separation results in us feeling stressed, confused, emotionally polarized, less than, more than, depressed, power hungry, victimized, anxious, and messy.

Messy personhood is dissonance in the mind. It's a personalized collection of habits, beliefs, resistance, stress, hang-ups, psychological trauma scars, emotional turbulence, and our struggle to remain curious and open. These facets arise from the parts of our mind that are divided and conflicted; they combine with our personality to create a unique signature of messiness. Our messy personhood has endless needs. It feels vulnerable and threatened and so lives in a state of fear and suffering, of aversion and craving—and then makes all that into a personal complex of problems.

Our messy personhood is most always looking for something to attach itself to, to define itself by, in order to uphold and strengthen its belief in its power and uniqueness as a separate self. One of the myriad of ways we do this is by attaching ourselves to our problems. This is why many of us find a large part of our sense of self intimately bound up with our problems—whether it's money, relationships, power, social status, security, fame or obscurity, body image, and so on. Most of what we call problems are our reaction to life simply unfolding around us, not to us or at us, as we often imagine. Note here that the mind itself is not dysfunctional; it's ready and teed up to be used as a wonderful tool. The messiness sets in when we confuse who we *are* with all of this mind-created perception of fear and suffering. This creates our messy personhood aspect of mind, which can take over our whole life and create significant unnecessary misery. Which can be a huge drag.

The only way out of this closed loop—to see ourselves more clearly—is to step outside the mind and observe it. To become the observer of our mind. Our inner **observer** is a bad-ass friend and supporter of awareness. Our observer self has no emotions, no judgment, no criticism, they only watch and reflect, like a mirror, exactly what they see. Our inner observer helps us more objectively see all the messy personhood stuff and then how those thoughts intermix to influence and create our experience of the world around us. What we experience on a moment-to-moment basis is a highly subjective existence—versus a factual, unfiltered experience of what's really out there. In other words, our internal state—our state of mind—is what determines our life experience, *not* the other way around. This is an important point, so I'm going to restate it another way. In the same way that putting a different lens in a camera changes what we see, our mind changes how we perceive our life experience.

And *this* is why it's life-changing to inquire into what's going on in our minds, because we're able to change our life experience by tending our mind. Change your mind, change your life. The more we *observe* our messy personhood, the less control it has over us. And the more we evolve the observer part of our consciousness, the more beautiful—and less messy—our existence becomes, and the more we find acceptance of our remaining messiness as we evolve. This observing creates increasing levels of health, joy, and personal evolution—a delightful, sometimes challenging, and precious life experience. In the next four sections, we'll explore the four main mind nemeses that keep us from that kind of experience, namely: resistance, emotional turbulence, stress turbulence, and trauma. We'll then learn the Ten Healing Practices for our mind and how to use them. Let's dig in.

Resistance, Revealed

Resistance is the central thread in why we're unhappy and unwell; it creates emotional turbulence and stress turbulence. Resistance is simply our internal railing against what *is*. It's akin to stepping onto a train track, seeing a train coming at us, and then complaining about the train being on the track, fretting that it's coming too fast, wondering why the conductor doesn't stop the train, being mad and judgmental toward the conductor, being pissed that trains can't stop more quickly—and not doing anything to move out of the way.

This may sound ridiculous, but it's how we live our lives: mentally resisting what is. Not only do we create our suffering with this resistance, we're completely missing the is-ness of the moment, which is that we're on a train track, where trains drive, and we're going to get squished if we don't move. Railing (pun intended) against the oncoming train is silly and a waste of our time and precious energy. This mental resistance can take a simple life event and turn it into full-on suffering. By resisting our experience, we're resisting ourselves. Most of us spend much of our lives in this stressful, emotionally charged mental state of resisting ourselves and everything around us.

Our resistance holds us back from fully living—from building a vibrant physical vehicle (body); tending a calm and powerfully connected mind; and living in alignment with the only part of us that's truly *us*, our spirit. But acceptance of what is often seems even scarier; hence, our most habitual and natural state is one of resistance and of not being fully committed to right now, because we're resisting what is.

When the mind is clear, we embrace what is, in the current moment. If we want the current reality to be different than it is, we might as well try to teach a bird to moo—it's not going to happen, and trying is going to make us suffer.

The vast majority of the stress we feel is caused by our internal argument with what is. In Buddhist philosophy, this resistance manifests via two sides of that same coin—craving and aversion. We have *aversion* to how things are, like railing against being stuck in traffic when we are stuck in traffic; and we *crave* how we want things to be, like wishing we were thinner when, in the moment, we're overweight. Both are resistance to what is. It's not life's circumstances that are causing emotional drama or stress, it's our resistance to life's circumstances. This is where personal responsibility is helpful. It allows us to own how we're using our mind, see that we're creating our unhappiness, and choose something different.

Note that our exploration of resistance *does not* mean that what's happening in the moment is something we necessarily want to promote, support, or continue. Our acceptance of reality doesn't mean we don't deal with things and make intentional moves toward change or improvement going forward. We do all that, for sure. We simply do it *in response* to what is—events that are continually taking place in our life experience—as opposed to *in reaction* to events and people that we feel are aiming to make us, personally, miserable. Reaction happens impulsively, quickly, and often with magnified emotion; a response is when we allow that reaction to happen inside ourselves, allow space to depersonalize and integrate, and then mindfully and intentionally move forward with verbal reply or action. We'll come to see that in the vast majority of situations, resistance is tied up in our fears and desires. Recognizing this allows us to dial down the drama and be present. It means that we see things without resistance and without the confusion of our inner struggle, which then frees us up to *act*. No one wants to be overweight; no one wants cancer; no one wants to be stuck in traffic; and no one wants to get fired. Yet our wish to be in a right-sized body, happy, employed, and disease-free does not always line up with our current reality; and it's not helpful, healing, or in any way volitional to mentally argue with what is. Even though I mentioned some ideas from Buddhist philosophy, this is not a philosophical or spiritual discussion. It's simply painful, in our mind, to argue with reality. Life is continually changing, and if we're constantly trying to control it, we'll never be able to fully live it; and not fully living our lives is, for many of us, sucking the joy out of our precious time here on Earth.

I invite you to stop for a moment and think about the impossible task that we've given our mind to do. We tell our mind: *"I want everyone to like me. I don't want anyone to speak badly of me. I want everything I say and do to be acceptable and pleasing to everyone. I don't want anyone to hurt me. I want to have everything I want, and nothing that I don't want. I don't want anything to happen that I don't like. And I want everything to happen that I do like."* Then we say to our mind: *"Now, figure out how to make every one of these things a reality, even if you have to think about it twenty-four hours a day."*

This inner conversation is at the heart of our enmeshed relationship with resistance, and why the mind is so active—we give it an impossible job to do. The simple antidote to our resistance is understanding that everything will be okay as soon as we are okay with everything. If that last sentence annoyed the snot out of you, I can assure you that it annoyed me the first time it came up for me, too. Why? Because this "simple" antidote goes against everything that we've trained our mind to do. Keeping my attention loosely on it over time, while cultivating curiosity in my mind, has shown it to be true and helpful, and thus slightly less annoying. The ancient text the *Bhagavad Gita* advises us: "The man who is self-controlled, who meets the objects of the senses with neither craving nor aversion, will attain serenity at last."

What we come to see is that pain is inevitable and suffering is optional. Pain and suffering are different things in this context. **Pain** happens in the moment, and **suffering** is a dragged-out mental exercise that is in direct opposition to equanimity and inner peace. Imagine what we might be capable of if our awareness was free to focus only on what is. So much of the noise, anxiety, and angst that continually take up space in our mind would subside. If we could bring this level of awareness and clarity to everything we do, our life experience would improve and our capabilities would be greater. It certainly won't happen overnight, but freeing our mind from this suffering and illusion is a key part of unlocking our potential. We can start by creating a practice of using daily life—the events that comprise our minute-by-minute, day-by-day experience—to let go of our resistance. Relationships are one of the best ways to work with ourselves. Imagine if we used relationships to get to know other people and ourselves, rather than to protect, satisfy, and defend what's blocked inside of us.

Surrender is the antidote to resistance. Surrender is one of those words—akin to compassion, vulnerability, and humility—that has been twisted in the cultural lexicon to denote a form of weakness. On the contrary, surrender is pivotal in our ability to inhabit a Creator Mindset, cultivate inner peace, live a vibrant life, and more fully express our spirit aspect. Surrender, in this context, is not resignation, nor is it non-action. It's not, *"Oh, I'm stuck in the mud, I guess I'll just stay here."* Surrender is not apathy or resistance or weakness. There's tremendous authentic power in surrender.

"Ugh, this makes no sense. I don't get it. If I always just give in to the way things are, I'm not going to make any effort to improve or change them. It's like when one army surrenders to another, 'We've given up. White flag. You win.'"

I know; the idea of surrender can seem like a turn-off. It's important to move past the military version of surrender involving white flags and heads hung in defeat, to consciously open to a different version. It's a tiny but powerful shift from seeing surrender as giving up, to grounding it in rock-solid empowerment. **Surrender** is relinquishing *our attachment* to the outcome. It's about not resisting this tiny little segment of time called the present: what IS. Surrender is the simple and profound wisdom of yielding to, rather than resisting, the flow of life in this moment, unconditionally and without reservation. We acknowledge, accept, and move on. Note that moving on can absolutely include damage control, taking action, initiating change, pursuing goals, and the like. Surrender is a different animal from an oh-well-who-cares attitude—that's resignation. If we look closely at the attitude of resignation, we'll find hidden resentment or apathy, which is actually veiled resistance.

When we surrender to the present, and then mindfully take positive action, it's far more effective than the negative action that arises out of anger, fear, despair, panic, or frustration. Once again, it's less about what we do and more about how we do it. Through surrender to the present moment, the quality of our consciousness, and, therefore, the quality and intention of whatever we're doing, becomes more powerful. We focus not on the forty-seven things that we believe need to happen this week, but on the one thing that we can do right now.

We don't have control over the future. When we think we have things all figured out and are attached to our little corner of knowledge and personal experience, we become closed to alternatives. We become unteachable. On the other hand, *"I don't know"* is an empowering statement that sets us up for curiosity and learning. Surrender allows us to relinquish our attachment to outcome, and become more mindful of how we *are* as we move toward the outcome we think we desire. We become focused on the internal journey as opposed to the external one. We invest fully in the moment-by-moment actions we take, the thoughts that we generate, and our intentions.

The power of surrender—taking action, and releasing our attachment to outcome—is a main thread throughout the *Bhagavad Gita*:

"You have a right to your actions, but never to your actions' fruits. Act for the action's sake."

. . . and . . .

"The wise man lets go of all results, whether good or bad, and is focused on the action alone."

These excerpts show us that surrender doesn't mean that we don't want what we're moving toward; it means that we're open to the idea that something else might be better for us, in the end. Surrender. That how we live our life, as opposed to where we're trying to get, is what's important. As the *Gita* says, " . . . *and best of all is surrender, which soon brings peace.*"

Surrender leads to freedom, and there are many shapes and sizes that surrender can come in. Resistance leads to suffering, and the forms of suffering are endless. Let's explore the three main forms of mental suffering—emotional turbulence, stress turbulence, and trauma—and their antidotes of emotional savvy, becoming stress-wise, and softening trauma.

Emotional Savvy

Emotions are a misunderstood part of our life experience, and our confusion about their nature and purpose can cause serious turbulence in our daily lives. If a being from another planet came to Earth and spent a day watching our news shows, reading social media, and eavesdropping on conversations, they would likely come to the conclusion that the human race is addicted to emotion. In the same way that we prop ourselves up with caffeine to start our day and then use evening alcohol to numb the business and stress of our day, we use emotions not only as entertainment but also as validation of our existence: I emote, therefore I am. We've become so wrapped up in our violence, our polarity, our desires, and our drama that we've lost sight of how it feels to be in equanimity. Emotions can be painful, draining, and all-consuming when used to entertain and define ourselves and our experience. This relationship with our emotions also allows marketers, newscasters, politicians, and all kinds of leaders and influencers to control us via our emotions. Yet, emotions are powerful, important, and useful when used as a tool to help guide us in the moment, assisting us in exploring and enjoying our life experience.

What are emotions, anyway? **Emotions** are currents of specific Energies, each with their own frequency, character, movement, and use. They're a communication that's first felt—if we pay attention—in the body, and then processed with our mind.

Emotional Energy, used mindfully, has the potential to help us protect ourselves, to heal, and to fully live the authentic expression of our unique selves. There's a part of our nonconscious mind that works with emotion beyond this initial instructive impulse, beyond the radar of our conscious mind.

Our emotions are a navigation system. They let us know when we need to move toward or away from a choice, person, or situation. In this way, they're a powerful force for enhancing our alignment and integration, within our BodyMindSpirit and relationally.

Our conscious mind provides a forum where we can actively process and learn from our helpful emotional messengers. However, this also means that we can use that conscious mind forum to hang on to an uncomfortable emotion for hours, weeks, or years—reliving it, magnifying its intensity, and painting our personal reality with its color. This is how emotional turbulence is created. While positive emotions like happiness can feel good, challenging emotions such as anger, jealousy, self-criticism, psychological fear, rejection, sadness, and loneliness can be difficult to navigate. As is often the case, it's our relationship to something that makes it good or bad, helpful or harmful, joyful or painful. Our relationship to challenging emotional Energy creates the turbulence, not the emotions themselves.

Most of us, much of the time, are wholly caught up in our unexamined emotional *reactions* to life. This, in turn, often lures us into the Victim Mindset, where we mistakenly believe that other people and circumstances are responsible for our joy and pain. We're lured into the social belief that life happens to us and at us, personally. It can certainly feel easier in the moment to believe this than to believe the truth. Yet in the final analysis, when our minds are able to be conscious observers, we know other people simply do or say things, events just happen, and then we feel emotions—*our* emotions.

I recently saw a quip that highlighted this idea: "Was it a bad day? Or was it a bad five minutes that you milked all day?" Most of us, myself included, have done our share of milking it, creating emotional turbulence. We feel an emotion and then we move into denial, drama (emoting with and onto others), or repression. We define ourselves, and the world around us, with our emotions. This doesn't mean we're idiots; it's simply our point of evolution with the mind. However, this unnecessary self-created emotional turbulence causes unhappiness and relational disaster—for people, organizations, and

countries. Maybe we're ready to stop the madness and evolve toward a different relationship with emotion.

Our relationship with emotions is similar to our relationship with physical
symptoms. A symptom is a messenger from our body to our mind that there's
imbalance that needs to be addressed. The symptom isn't what needs fixing, the
functional imbalance is. For instance, as mentioned earlier, we often take painkillers (Advil, Tylenol, aspirin) when we get a headache. Many headaches are
caused by chronic dehydration. Yet, in the case of chronic dehydration, instead
of giving our body water in response to our symptom of a headache, we numb
the headache with painkillers, while the imbalance of dehydration continues
and worsens. When we suppress physical symptoms with painkillers or other
pharmaceuticals, the foundational issue is left untouched and will continue to
become more imbalanced. This leads to continued and escalated dysfunction
and suffering rather than balance and healing.

When we react to the messages of our emotions, it's often the same deal.
We tend to ignore them, suppress them, or project them onto others, rather
than honoring them as part of our GPS and getting busy with our curiosity
around what we need to move toward or away from. The journey from emotional drama, confusion, and the personalization of all that we encounter—to
equanimity—is challenging because our culture (and therefore each one of us)
is deeply conflicted about our emotions. A central piece of that inner conflict
is that we have the illusion that we *are* our emotions—that in some way they
define us. This idea adds to our emotional turbulence, and we've become so
enmeshed with emotion-gone-amuck that we've lost our perspective. The great
news is, we can reduce this turbulence by better using the tool of mind.

EMOTION AS A TOOL

Developing emotional savvy—better known as emotional intelligence—is a
key aspect of creating the life experience that we desire. Emotional intelligence—also called EI or EQ ("Q" for Quotient)—is an idea that was defined

by researchers and psychologists Drs. Peter Salovey and John Mayer (not the singer) and popularized by psychologist and journalist Daniel Goleman in *Emotional Intelligence*. **Emotional intelligence** encompasses intrapersonal (within ourselves) and interpersonal (between us and someone else) emotional savvy. It's our ability, along a continuum, to be aware of, navigate, and express emotions. Here, we're exploring intrapersonal EQ; in Chapter 10, we'll dive into interpersonal EQ.

The first and most important step is to understand emotions for what they are. Emotions represent a shift in our nonphysical integration; they are an important tool in our internal navigation system, functioning as messengers. Learning to heed these emotional messengers will support you in incorporating emotions—the very ones you feel each day—as part of your path toward the fullness of you. Emotions get us closer to our truth than thinking can, if we can *intentionally engage* with them rather than getting caught up in them, reacting to them, and creating drama for ourselves and others. Emotions simply need to have their day in the sun—to be acknowledged, honored, and released—in order to function in their key role in navigating life and encouraging integration and wholeness.

The pure emotion as felt in the body is completely truthful—sometimes painfully so—and is rife with opportunities for healing. Between stimulus and response—between emotion-as-messenger and our words or actions—we have the freedom to choose. When we move into the reactive state that we've been discussing, we become the emotion. When we see emotion as a message that we can be guided by and respond to, our personal responsibility helps us to choose thoughts, words, and actions that will positively influence the future of our lives, our society, and our planet. This type of intentional response to the impulse of an emotion's message helps us to integrate our whole-person experience, to grow our self-worth, and to expand and deepen our self-care. This ability to intentionally respond paves the way to reducing chronic stress, better understanding our life experience, cultivating healthier relationships, and embodying authentic living. Good stuff.

It's also hard. The reason that emotional drama, denial, or repression can be so damaging is that emotions carry massive amounts of Energy with them. We've all felt the power of emotions, and the idea of responding instead of reacting can sound almost impossible. Further, many of our habits and behaviors—programmed in our formative years—affect the way we emotionally react. Between this old wiring and the powerful force behind emotion, intentionally shifting our relationship with our emotions ends up being a lifelong practice for most of us.

YOUR EMOTIONS ARE YOUR EMOTIONS

When we listen carefully to the conversations that go on in the world around us, that go on in our lives, and that transpire inside our head, an interesting common thread appears. We often blame our emotions on other people—we say that someone *made* us feel a certain way. Then, we label the person who "made us" feel that way as difficult, mean, inconsiderate, and the like. Those labels may or may not be true, but the truth is that no one can make us feel anything. *Our emotions are our emotions.* Someone can say or do something that we don't appreciate, but they can't control how we feel—only we control that. Thus, flexing our personal responsibility muscles is key to emotional health, balance, and integration.

Let's examine a lens through which our view of "difficult people" can be changed forever, a lens that helps us see our emotions more clearly. Jōsei Toda, the late Japanese teacher, peace activist, and revolutionary thinker, suggested that we imagine ourselves as glasses of water. Next, we imagine that our past negative experiences, our preferences, and our messy personhood is soil in the bottom of our glass. Another person comes along and acts as a spoon, stirring up the soil that we already had in our glass. They didn't put the soil in there; they stirred what was already there. If there were no soil in the bottom of our glass, there'd be nothing to swirl up (emotions) and cloud our water. Therefore, the foundational issue isn't other people, it's that we need to identify our soil and put our intention on sifting some of it out of our glass.

This important insight deeply shifted the way I process my challenging emotions. Toda taught that if something upsets us, the first step is self-examination, because the same words or actions that can trigger one person to become upset may leave another completely unfazed. Therefore, the emotions (the swirling soil) can be attributed only to ourselves, not to others. Our emotions are wholly ours.

This was an awakening for my client Alisha—first an uncomfortable one, then an empowering one. My work with Alisha was largely focused on helping her postmenopausal body come back to balance, with the intent of reigniting her metabolism. She felt sluggish and overweight. Some key areas we were exploring were food and beverages, sleep, movement, hormones, herbal support, and psychological stress. Chronic negative emotions are stressors and Alisha shared with me that one of her employees, whom she found challenging, continually took her power away. This relationship was a source of constant stress for her.

Me: "Well, I understand that Brad is challenging for you, but he can't take your power away."

Alisha: "Yes he can. He does it all the time."

Me: "Bear with me here, Alisha, but the question that's coming up for me is, why are you giving your power away to Brad?"

Alisha: "I'm not. He's a jerk and he gets defensive and combative whenever I bring up something that needs to be changed or done differently."

Me: "Right. Alisha, Brad's just Brad. And you're his boss. What is it about Brad that brings up feelings of powerlessness for you? Where are you not having good boundaries?"

Alisha was quiet for quite a few seconds after that. It was hard to not continue talking, but I sensed she was having an "aha" moment and making an important self-discovery. After a pause, she understood and got excited about the idea that Brad, or anyone else for that matter, wasn't the driver of her emotional bus. She had come to the understanding that her emotions are her emotions.

"But what about those of us who are just super sensitive and feel like their feelings are always getting run over by others?"

Yes, there are many of us who are true **sensitives**—folks who have more depth of processing, are more easily overstimulated, are more sensitive to subtleties in our environment, and feel emotions more strongly than the average bear. Highly sensitive people fall into an estimated 20 percent of the population, as researched by psychologist Elaine Aron. This is different than being easily offended. Many of us who call ourselves sensitive are instead covertly self-absorbed; constantly struggling with worry, insecurity, and defensiveness while holding on to the view that other people's words and actions happen *to* us, as opposed to simply happening.

I know that can sound a bit harsh. However, the reality is, if we focus on how everything is making *us* feel, as opposed to taking responsibility for our emotions and becoming curious about other people, then we're thinking about ourselves an awful lot. And, we may be wanting other people to change in order to compensate for our messy personhood. This approach is not the one that leads to joy.

It's important that we all—all 7.6 billion of us—remember that our emotions get brought up by our stuff, our soil at the bottom of our glass. When we take responsibility for our emotional state, we set the stage for relating to others from a place of empowerment and clarity. This leads to us feeling more comfortable with who we are, and to no longer need other people to validate us and tell us we're okay. We won't get comfortable with ourselves as long as we're blaming our emotions on other people and circumstances. Our self-worth, that important pillar in our health and well-being, will most always suffer.

The trick is that emotions are powerful and can feel uncomfortable, and we're neurologically wired to avoid discomfort. This means that leaning into uncomfortable emotions has to be an intentional *act*. It rarely happens on its own, but it's the only way to clear the way for understanding. The philosopher Baruch Spinoza said, "The more clearly you understand yourself and your emotions, the more you become a lover of what is." This relates directly back to our exploration of resistance. Resistance is fuel for the fire of emotional drama. The more we allow initial emotional hits to instruct us in the moment—to move toward or away from something—the more comfortable we become with ourselves, with others, and with the often-difficult realities of the world around us. Life is beautiful *and* challenging.

Our daily emotions are best met with awareness. When we welcome them from a place of compassion, and acknowledge that it's more than okay—indeed, important—to notice and feel our emotions, we learn to let go of our need to control our lives and experiences. Pushing our everyday emotions aside hinders our ability to integrate our experiences and causes disruptions in our inner balance. In the same way that the GPS in our car will keep working to reroute us if we dismiss its route suggestions and get farther off track, our dismissed emotions will continue to pop up in an effort to guide us.

I encourage you to process your emotions via discussion or journaling. The simple act of journaling—writing down thoughts—can help provide insight and perspective into our mind and emotions. It provides a forum where we can ask ourselves guiding questions about our emotions to gain insight into their messages. What wants to be released? What wants to be restored? Where am I moving into chaos or rigidity in my mind? What helps me feel aligned? Do I hang on to my opinions and preferences (clinging) or do I let go? Where am I allowing judgment to color my perspective of reality? What must be protected? Where am I not being honest with myself?

Where do I need boundaries? Where do I have unnecessary barriers? What action(s) need(s) to be taken?

Ideally, we'll begin to notice the emotion and then get curious about where our life experience is becoming more or less aligned. What is it that we want to move toward, or away from? The *I Ching,* the ancient Chinese divination *Book of Changes,* reads, "It is only when we have the courage to face things exactly as they are, without any self-deception or illusion, that a light will develop out of events, by which the path to success may be recognized." Untended challenging emotions can significantly muddy the waters of our reality; they are ripe for creating self-deception and relational discord. Therefore, mindfully working with them is an instructive and courageous path.

If we're not intimate with our all-important emotional messengers, then we can't pick up on the dynamics that lie beneath them or the integration and healing they exist to serve. Awareness of these strong currents of Energy is the first step in learning how our daily experiences come into being and why. Awareness also helps us to begin honoring our emotions and supporting their flow. It's that very flow that opens our heart and invites healing. Cultivating these aspects of our lives is more of a meditation; meaning, it's an intention that we practice each day, knowing that it won't be perfect. The good news is that it's the process that's important. Health, joy, and personal evolution are not linear, nor are they a destination that we reach. Infusing mindfulness and intention into our emotional lives allows us to shift how our emotions affect us personally, as well as how they contribute to the world around us. In addition to the inherent value of cultivating emotional savvy, this skill also helps us reduce chronic stress.

Becoming Stress-Wise

The past fifty years have seen stress become a top barrier to our well-being. Each day, we turn everyday setbacks, challenges, and busyness into stress and overwhelm. Our species' evolution over 200,000 years has not accommodated for this abrupt change in our response to the complexities of life. Each year, new research and warnings are published that link chronic stress to chronic disease and mental dysfunction.

We seem to have created an entire culture based on the cultivation and worship of stress, couched in an underlying fear—of what, we're not certain. Our way-back ancestors had real use for fear and its associated physiological reactions; then it was about survival and fear was instructive and often life-saving. Here in the twenty-first century, we're not facing the same threats, such as predators or an attacking tribe suddenly appearing over the hill. Instead, we live with *psychological fear*, which begets *psychological stress*. But let's not get ahead of ourselves. What is stress? Is stress bad? What does it mean to be stressed out? How does stress impact our health, our mind, and our ability to create inner peace and equanimity?

It's important to first define stress in order to open our eyes to what's truly going on with stress and our well-being. *Stress* was originally a physics term defined as "a pressure, pull, or force exerted on one material object by another." When I sit in a chair, the force of my weight being pulled by gravity creates stress in the structure of the chair (and in my butt, which is why it gets sore after a while). We took that physics term and applied it to our mental life, where our *perception* of demanding or adverse external events and circumstances creates pressure or tension on our mind.

If the perceived adversity is an extremely short-term event, such as being grabbed by a mugger or seeing an oncoming car veer into our driving lane, this reaction is **survival stress**. With this kind of stress, the related biochemical and neurological responses in our body can be helpful and life-saving. If the adversity is an important meeting that we're preparing for over a matter of days or weeks, the heightened energy and drive that results from those related biochemical and neurological responses can assist us *if our inner approach is positive and can-do.* This differentiating inner approach moves us into **challenge stress**, where we view a challenging circumstance as something that can help us grow, as opposed to something that might take us down at the knees.

However, the type of stress that most of us suffer from on a daily basis is **psychological stress**, when the perceived challenges are not life-threatening at all, but we still feel threatened, overwhelmed, and helpless. These circumstances that we perceive as stressors might include: a colleague whom we find personally challenging; a leaky roof; a company culture that isn't aligned with our personal values; a sick family member; a traffic jam; work and family life balance; budget issues; a long to-do list; or world politics. The list is long and, unfortunately, our biochemistry and resulting neurological and physiological responses are exactly the same whether the perceived adversity is a mugger or a traffic jam.

Going forward, when I use the word *stress*, I'll be referring to psychological stress, unless I note otherwise. You may have noticed my frequent use of the word *perceived*. The word *perceived* is pivotal to this discussion, as all stress results from perceived adversity. This tiny point—this single word—is where the whole crux of our stress issues reside. Psychological studies have been done where subjects are shown images and their stress levels are recorded via a device similar to a polygraph machine. If an image of a dog is shown, the majority of people don't register a stress response, because lots of people like dogs and feel comfortable with them. However, if that participant had been attacked by a dog, especially recently, they might perceive the dog image as threatening, and that image would evoke a stress response in them. What one person perceives as a threat, the other might not. Further, what one person perceives as a threat on one day might barely register as a problem on another day for that same person.

If I get stuck in a traffic jam on a Monday evening on my way to go food shopping, I might simply chill out and listen to music. If I get stuck in a traffic jam again on Wednesday morning on my way to catch a flight at the airport, I might go into full stress response. A traffic jam on one day is cause to chill out, while a traffic jam less than forty-eight hours later is cause to freak out. Why? Because modern-day stress is largely a mind-created phenomenon, predicated entirely on perception. The trick is, our physiological reaction is the same, regardless if the "threat" is real or imagined.

THE SCIENCE OF STRESS

When our mind perceives threat or adversity, our brain activates our sympathetic nervous system, which in turn activates our fight-or-flight response. We can think of the sympathetic nervous system as the gas pedal in our car. In less than a second (nerve impulses can travel up to 390 feet per second), our perception of adversity triggers our hypothalamus, a tiny control-center gland in our brain. The hypothalamus elicits a cascade of hormones with far-reaching effects. Biochemically, this involves an influx of hormones such as cortisol and adrenaline; and an increase in blood sugar, which prompts an influx of insulin. In the case of chronic stress, these sustained hormonal changes pull other hormones out of balance and deeply affect how our body functions. Looking at the stress response from a physiology standpoint, blood flow is being shunted away from digestion, reproduction, and other nonimmediate survival systems while dramatic increases in heart rate, respiratory rate, and muscle energy and tension occur. This is all fabulous and helpful if we've run into a mugger or have stumbled across a mother bear in the woods with her cubs—not so fabulous or helpful if we're constantly stressed about everyday life.

These changes help our body perform well for a true immediate emergency, priming our body for optimum strength and speed. For example, my seventh-grade English teacher, Mrs. Carter, was in a car accident in her twenties. There were four people in the car and the car was grotesquely totaled, trapping one guy in the back with a lit cigarette on the floor out of his reach. He started screaming about the cigarette and the gas tank.

She wrenched open the door and dragged him away from the car (it later turned out that he had a broken ankle and a concussion). When a police officer arrived, he examined the car and asked how the four of them had gotten the back door open. Mrs. Carter said she had opened it. The officer looked up and down her five-foot, tiny frame and declared it impossible. *"The hinges are mangled. The actual door is bent open. You would've had to bend steel with your bare hands. How did you really get it open?"* What he didn't know was that she'd also dragged out a 200-pound man. She'd been fueled by her powerful stress response and accomplished amazing feats that would normally have been impossible.

This powerful stress response is decidedly less amazing when triggered for chronic psychological stress. Over time, many areas of the body go into dysfunction as we overdose on a constant drip of sympathetic-driven chemical changes. Heartburn, cardiovascular damage, low fertility, adrenal fatigue, muscle tension and headaches, weight gain, exhastion, hypothyroidism, compromised digestion, cancer, high blood pressure, type 2 diabetes, insomnia, and immune suppression are some of the main physical effects linked to chronic stress. Mental effects include irritability, fatigue, depression, anxiety, and heightened emotional reactivity. The continual release of cortisol that accompanies chronic stress damages our brain. More recent research has even shown that chronic stress erodes our telomeres. Telomeres are handy little endcaps on our DNA strands that protect our DNA, in a similar way that the hard ends of shoelaces protect our laces from fraying. A great many alterations are made to the inner state and workings of our body as a result of chronic stress.

All of this is further proof of the power of thought, because psychological stress is caused by the *perception* of adversity. These thoughts create significant changes in our biochemistry and physiology, and science is only just beginning to understand their ramifications. Meanwhile, the general population has come to culturally accept chronic stress as normal, not understanding how detrimental and costly stress truly is. Chronic stress is common but not normal. Without pussy-footing around, chronic stress is a killer. If stress were a communicable disease, we'd be declaring ourselves in the midst of a plague and would be wildly working to find a cure.

MIND YOUR MINDSET

The double irony about chronic stress is that the cure is already available, *and* it comes from the same place that caused the dis-ease: our mind-brain. Chronic stress is an example of the mind acting as a barrier. It's the result of an unhealthy relationship between our mind and the forces perceived in our environment—and *it's our response to these forces*, as opposed to the forces themselves, that determines our outcome. Mark Twain said it well: "I've had a lot of worries in my life, most of which never happened." It's funny to read, but the reason his words are funny is that they ring with uncomfortable truth. Not only is most of our worrying about things outside of our circle of influence, but a majority of our worries never come to fruition. Yet many of us convince ourselves that our worry and anxiety does something to keep problems at bay. Moreover, if I'm a stressed-out person, then I will experience the world as a stressful place. I experience feelings of stress at work, at home, at the holidays, driving, in the market, getting dressed, or sitting on the beach. *I am* the creator of the stress, so I take it with me wherever I go. Hundreds of millions of people feel this way, to varying degrees. Our stress is not unique. Yet, we feel as if *our* life is particularly stressful and that we're uniquely stressed out.

Now it's time for a little tough love. When we hide behind the words *"stressed out,"* we're relinquishing our personal responsibility, making ourselves out to be some tiny, fragile boat on an illusory stormy ocean of stress. We short-change our ownership as the steward of a vibrant BodyMindSpirit vehicle and designate ourselves as victims—of schedules, deadlines, finances, personality clashes, work, illness, the weather, trauma, and life itself. And we tell everyone, all day, over and over, about the over-the-top difficulties and busyness of our lives. While the vast majority of us believe that stress lives out there and is out of our control, in actuality, stress lives "in here"—in our mind—and is completely within our control.

"That's ridiculous. I'm actually very busy for real and never have enough time, which constantly stresses me out."

You actually do have enough time. Let's unpack our relationship with time.

DECODING THE TYRANNY OF TIME

Time. I'm glad you brought it up. (Okay, okay; I brought it up.) Most of us complain to varying degrees about our lack of time. This complaint comes from our running on a stress hamster-wheel, which puts us on psychological time. **Psychological time** is different from clock time, in the same way that psychological fear is different from survival fear, and that psychological stress is different from survival stress. Clock time is real, while psychological time is mind-created and mixed up with emotions and psychological fear.

If I make a mistake today and actively process what happened, learning from it, then I am using clock time, which is the real deal. On the other hand, if I make a mistake today and then swirl into a mental dwelling-on and rehashing of my mistake—cultivating self-criticism, remorse, guilt, blame, and shame—then I've mentally made this mistake a part of my present sense of self. I've incorporated this past mistake into my messy personhood and have moved into psychological time. Nonforgiveness—of ourselves or of another—implies a heavy burden of psychological time, of living in a past heavily burdened with blame and regret. This is how psychological time adds to our stress burden.

In the more tactical realm, if I got fired and needed to find a job, I might work toward reemployment each day by setting aside a block of time when I engage in job-hunting activities. I'm using clock time. I'm aware that I want to end up employed in the future, but I'm largely focused on the present moment by giving my full attention to job-hunting tasks. However, if I instead gripe about the unfair way I was fired and worry about my age and the economy, while haphazardly asking around about employment opportunities, the present is no longer honored. I allow my lack of employment to suck the value out of the present moment. I've now shifted out of clock time and into psychological time. My BodyMindSpirit journey is no longer an adventure I'm present for; it's instead an obsessive chase after the fantasy of future security, perfection, attainment, or validation.

When we operate in psychological time, time becomes our ever-present persecutor and we fall into an endless loop of the Victim Mindset. It's this relationship with time and stress that's currently eroding our health, creating disease, challenging our relationships; and sucking the wonder, creativity, and joy out of our life experience. Our greatest tormentor is our untended mind. In the same way that our relationship to perceived stressors causes our issues (as opposed to the stressors themselves), it's our relationship with time that's an issue, not time itself.

Migrating our relationship with time—from psychological time to clock time—requires mindfulness and diligence. The basic approach is to flex our mighty personal responsibility muscle and catch ourselves when we complain about time, use it as an excuse, or jump into "I'm-so-much-busier-than-you" verbal competitions. This kind of awareness can be challenging, for sure, so I suggest you start with a micromovement by habitually making small changes to your dialogue, such as this:

Buying into psychological time:
Kid: Will you throw the football with me?
Dad: I don't have time.

vs.

Honoring clock time:

Kid: Will you throw the football with me?

Dad: I want to finish what I'm working on before we throw the football. I'll be ready to hang out with you in thirty minutes.

Do you hear and feel the difference? Moving more into clock time creates subtle, yet powerful, changes in our life experience. When we live with psychological fear and psychological time, we unconsciously distance ourselves from others, buying into a self-image of being special—better or worse, busier or more balanced, blessed or cursed—and this weakens our feeling of connection to all beings. In contrast, I've found that when someone is open-hearted and living more in clock time, they're most often relaxed. Or what my sons would call *chill.* Ever meet those folks who seem perpetually easygoing? We tell ourselves that maybe they're not as busy as we are, or our job is more important and demanding, or our kids are needier, or that we're special because we're the breadwinner for our family, or our financial situation is harder, or we're a single parent, or we face more challenges, and on and on. In truth, some people operate more in clock time than others; and they carry their easygoing approach wherever they go, regardless of challenges that pop up.

What these chill folks who live more in clock time have discovered is that modern life stressors can't be avoided. Our challenge—our opportunity—is deciding how we respond to them. A main antidote for feeling stressed out is changing our relationship with time, and continually tending to the balance in our life—creating time for family and friends; adequate nutrition, sleep, and rest; movement, play and laughter; and connection to our spiritual self through prayer, chanting, meditation, communing with nature, or whatever floats our boat. Balance will rarely be perfect or lasting—it's an ongoing adaptive process. We continually adapt to the circumstances in which we live. Contrary to what many pulled from Charles Darwin's *On the Origin of the Species*, it's *adaptability* to a changing environment that he emphasized as key to survival of species. Adaptability and resilience are where it's at. A cure for our chronic stress—for our mal-adapted way of responding to daily life—is changing our mind by utilizing stress-management tools, while developing stress resilience. Let's explore.

STRESS MANAGEMENT

Stress management consists of simple habits and tactics that we can practice in our everyday lives. Most of these tactics invoke a relaxation response from the parasympathetic nervous system (home of our "rest and digest" response), which opposes our chronic stress responses from the sympathetic nervous system (home of our "fight-or-flight" response). What is the **relaxation response**? It's when you sit in your La-Z-Boy recliner with a beer. Kidding! The relaxation response works to balance off stress hormones and neutralize them. We can think of the relaxation response as the brake in our car, offsetting daily stress accumulation and helping us to build stress resilience.

The relaxation response is a term coined by Herbert Benson, cardiologist, Harvard professor, and founder of the Benson-Henry Institute for Mind Body Medicine at Massachusetts General Hospital in Boston. The relaxation response promotes balance—in the moment and cumulatively over time—within our nervous system and our entire body. What can we actively do to invoke the relaxation response? I use the acronym BRETH to help me remember the tools that intercept the stress response and bring us back to being calm and empowered:

Breathing snack

Reset

Exercise burst

Time out

Happiness

A *breathing snack* is when we stop and take thirty seconds for three slow, deep breaths from our diaphragm, elongating the exhale. When you try this, put your hand on your belly to make sure it's moving in and out, which indicates that you're fully using your diaphragm, as opposed to using upper-chest breathing. You can do a breathing snack anywhere, anytime—at your work desk, waiting in line, sitting at a traffic light, sitting on scaffolding, sitting on the toilet, or lying in bed upon waking and before sleeping. Distributing breathing snacks throughout our day will put a wet blanket on the fires of stress, minimizing its effects on our body and mind. Breathing snacks provide a mini-relaxation response that can change your brain chemistry for the better.

Meditation, visualization, and spending time in nature can provide a mental *reset* and help you generate equanimity and joy. In using visualization, we close our eyes and visualize ourselves in a place where we feel relaxed—Aruba, the forest, our favorite lake or beach—and take careful notice of the minute details of that happy place, like smells, sounds, skin sensation, taste, and sights. With visualization, we're utilizing that aspect of the mind-brain that can't tell the difference between real and imagined—this time to our advantage. When our perception is that we're in our happy place, our whole physiology responds by relaxing. Time spent in nature tends to bring us into the present moment and we feel connected to things we are a part of—the natural world, which can invoke the relaxation response. Meditation, which we'll be covering toward the end of this chapter, is also a powerful inducer of the relaxation response and functions aptly in stress management and in creating stress resilience.

Other simple activities that you can combat daily stress with are a quick exercise burst, like running up and down stairs a few times; taking a time-out in a different environment; and writing down three to five things for which you're grateful, bringing about feelings of happiness and "can-do." In addition to helping us manage stress in the moment, these tactics also help us to build stress resilience. What is stress resilience and how is it different from stress management?

Metaphorically, let's say that the Wicked Witch of the West (WWotW) from *The Wizard of Oz*—one of my favorite characters—comes to me to discuss her fatal relationship with water. The WWotW is melted by water, so we're going to use water as our metaphor for stress.

I could tell the WWotW where all of the rain shelters are in her neighborhood. I could provide her with herbal healing remedies to unmelt if she happens to get caught in the rain. I could put an app on her smartphone that forecasts the weather for her, helping her to avoid rain (and then activate the app that doesn't let her check the weather while she's riding her broomstick, of course). I could familiarize her with what a hose and sprinkler systems look like, so she could avoid them. I could suggest that she purchase rain gear and keep it handy at all times. Important info, and useful for her, to navigate the water that may show up, and to help her avoid melting. These tips and precautions for the WWotW are similar to stress management techniques for us nonwitches.

Even better? I could provide her with a patented body lotion that she applies twice a year that makes water roll right off her skin. Then, she's freed from her fear of water and will rarely need the other tips, gear, and cool app, because her whole relationship to rain has changed. And for us mere humans, the equivalent to that patented body lotion, in the stress arena, is STRESS RESILIENCE.

STRESS RESILIENCE

Stress resilience refers to our ability to withstand and adapt to what we perceive as stressors and adverse events. We achieve this skill when we regain our innate ability to effectively cope with stressors and quickly return to equilibrium. This resilience means we need to cultivate a different relationship to self-care, to time, and to life events. Over time, many things that once felt stressful no longer have the same negative charge.

When we're resilient, for example, we might notice our breathing is shallow and that we feel anxious, that we've shifted into psychological fear. We can then take a deep, slow breath from our diaphragm and consciously reframe the current situation as life with all its inherent challenges. We can remind ourselves that we've handled everything up to now, and this will be no different. We could then ease our expectations that life should be easy and relinquish the idea that our life is particularly hard. Over time, as a result of these choices, we would spend more time in equanimity and come back to it more quickly when ruffled by a stressor.

The cultivation of stress resilience includes the ideas in this book—building personal responsibility and self-worth, practicing self-care, honoring our body, tending our mind, and living our Spirit. There are also some specific inner approaches that we can practice, which are the hallmarks of resilience. Resilience is something we embody, rather than something we do, although it's important to understand that stress-management tactics can help us build stress resilience.

Like many worthwhile things, stress resilience is simple in concept but takes time and care to develop. I like to remember them by saying, *"I will develop Mi PECs"*:

Mindfulness

Perception

Emotional **I**ntelligence

Creator Mindset

The first stress-resilience practice is *mindfulness*. We touched on mindfulness as one of the Three Amigos; we'll also be exploring it more fully at the end of this chapter. As a reminder, mindfulness is open, active attention to the present moment, without judgment. It creates stress resilience by bringing us squarely into the present and away from our stories—our perceptions—about the alleged future ramifications of our stressful-feeling situation.

Perception is a key word in the definition of stress. Because stress is a result of *perceived* adversity, as we develop more intention and focus in our mind, we can shift our perception. We can conduct a stress reappraisal. For instance, let's say our car runs out of gas. We often habitually react to this type of scenario from a place of psychological fear. We tell ourselves futuristic stories about being late to a meeting or about the danger of the area where our car is disabled. We could delve into the past, focusing on how stupid we were to not fill the tank. We react in these ways that don't serve either us or the situation. We're generating needless stress hormones over a non-survival-related life situation.

Instead, as we build our stress resilience, we're able to take a few breaths and intentionally shift our perception in a way that is more realistic and doesn't negatively affect our BodyMindSpirit health. *Slow, deep breath. Slow, deep breath. Okay, although this is not ideal, it's really just an inconvenience. No one, including me, will die because I ran out of gas. What actions can I take to respond to what IS: me, in a car, out of gas?* This simple exercise is a game-changer. Getting perspective and giving yourself a reality check stops the stress response in its tracks.

Emotional intelligence is another important tool for developing stress resilience. As we just explored, EQ helps us to be aware of and utilize our emotional messengers in a way that supports happiness, growth, and interconnection. We become empowered around our emotions, as opposed to feeling that people and events outside of ourselves are creating them. Feelings of empowerment create stress resilience; feelings of powerlessness do not.

The *Creator Mindset* is important for all aspects of our life journey, including developing stress resilience. Psychological stress arises from mental stories that have their roots in victimhood. A traffic jam, a disturbing health report, our struggling child, our lack of time, our financial challenges, the long line we're waiting in, our demanding job, our difficult spouse, and life in general are not all conspiring against us. They simply are. When we put ourselves in the Victim Mindset, we are the ones conspiring against ourselves by giving away our powers. Our powers of intention, problem solving, response, and equanimity, to name a few. The Creator Mindset is a powerful ally in developing stress resilience. The size of the stressor doesn't matter; it's our capacity and willingness to respond mindfully that counts.

Why is it so important to learn stress resilience? Other than all of the physical and mental reasons we just covered? When we feel stressed out, we're disconnected from our flow, agility, creativity, sense of humor, instincts, intuition, and ability to set boundaries. Our perspective becomes narrow and laser-focused on our trials and tribulations, which causes further stress when we lose sight of the big picture. Stress resilience turns down the volume on that bumpin' bass in our mind that frames everything as a cause for worry.

Stress resilience hinges on us becoming a more conscious steward of our mind. It's learning that we have emotions, but we're not those emotions. It's created by becoming adept at reframing our perspective so that we can reduce the Victim Mindset, and therefore reduce psychological stress. It's about changing our relationship with time. Over time, we'll find that we get stressed-out far less than we used to; we become resilient to psychological stress.

Our life experience becomes more relaxed, focused, and connected, as we are freed up to live with the passion, joy, and purpose that we were born with. Over time, we'll develop an inner peace that permeates our entire life experience and supports our BodyMindSpirit health. We've explored two of the top three forms of mental suffering—emotional turbulence and stress turbulence—and uncovered how we can utilize our mind to heal suffering and support our personal evolution. And this conversation on mind health and integration would not be complete without shining a light on the third main form of mental suffering: trauma.

Softening Trauma: "Sit with Your Shit"

We touched on trauma briefly earlier, and it's worth a closer look. Think about surviving a car accident—you may still be alive, but you'd have some degree of physical trauma—cuts, bruises, broken bones, whiplash, concussion, and/or internal bleeding. Similarly, psychological **trauma** is damage to the psyche as a result of any type of mind-brain or physical stimulus that, in its intensity, sends a person hurtling away from themselves—into *dissociation*.

Dissociation is a protective reaction of the mind—where a person disconnects from their thoughts, feelings, memories, or even their sense of identity—most often in response to trauma. This can occur due to many types of events, including molestation, rape and sexual abuse, physical abuse, emotional head games, cruelty, neglect, abandonment, painful surgeries, hospitalizations, scary dental work, accidents, witnessing a terrible event, or even getting trapped in an elevator. Sometimes, in the very young especially, trauma-induced dissociation is so complete that the trauma is stored in implicit memory, which means it can't be recalled at will. This creates a major barrier for healing. Reflexive dissociation is a powerful and necessary survival skill in the moment. The real damage is not in the immediate danger, or in the dissociation in the moment, but in the fact that we don't have the resilience to re-embody our integrated sense of self once the danger has passed.

Trauma survivors can continue to see danger where danger doesn't exist, long after the dangerous events cease. Life itself can become traumatizing. The heart of the trauma survivor can become blocked by these stored, highly detailed, unfinished Energy patterns from the past. Sadly, the blocked heart of the traumatized, along with the dissociation that accompanies trauma, often leads them to act out trauma again and again, traumatizing themselves or traumatizing others. They can feel deep shame, and the feelings of shame can become a habitual way of seeing themselves. These patterns may be held within trauma survivors for a long time, and can quietly or not-so-quietly run their lives, developing into a complex core of suffering that also ripples out to those around them.

Let's get something out of the way that will allow us to look at the important subject of trauma through the lens of reality: almost everyone has some level of trauma from childhood. Most of us were bullied, teased, abused, neglected, or mistreated by the people in our environment—parents, siblings, relatives, neighbors, religious or spiritual leaders, teachers, bosses, co-workers, coaches, or peers—or have experienced other traumatizing events. Family life is a major source of trauma, as the whole family thing can be *pretty messy*. In families, we don't have only one messy personhood carrying trauma, emoting and resisting what is; we have several people all interacting with one another. Our parents—as flawed people navigating their own belief systems, programming, trauma, pain, and confusion—were operating in parenthood without an instruction manual, sometimes angry, confused, and self-centered, like all people. This doesn't mean that what they did as parents was always okay, or that they or we are excused from bad behavior; it simply means that screwing up—along a wide continuum—is part of the territory. Meanwhile, traumatic experiences can shape who we are, emotionally, neurobiologically, and physically. Via the triple interplay of biology and neurochemistry and mind, trauma doesn't just change our belief systems and our behavior, our genetic material can also be altered by trauma. There's only one way out of this storm: confronting our pain by sitting with it.

Occupational therapist Kim Barthel, a thought leader in the areas of trauma, addiction, and healing, wrote in *Conversations with a Rattlesnake* that the way through trauma is to "sit with our shit." When we have unaddressed trauma, we often desperately seek ways to shellac over our dissociated pain—to cover up our shit. This is the genesis of addiction, in all its forms. Each addiction arises from an unconscious refusal to face and move through our pain. Eventually our addiction reaches a point where it doesn't work for us anymore, and then we feel the pain more intensely than ever. The pain has been growing and morphing under the shellac, and it's breaking through in an amped-up effort to win our attention. The only way out of this intense pain is through it, which means sifting out and feeling the painful feelings that we tried to avoid, facing layers of shame and pain. In other words, we sit with our shit. This is a necessary and painful step to healing but, as Rumi suggested in his poem "Childhood Friends," our wound is the place where the Light enters us.

Most of us, however, don't take this unhealed trauma as a place where grace or healing can enter. Psychological wounds can be a source of significant discomfort. Generally speaking, we regard discomfort in any form as bad news, and there's no discomfort like the red-hot mess at the heart of unhealed trauma. We're mentally focused on running from the pain of the trauma, which makes sense because we're neurologically wired to escape pain and seek pleasure. So we run like crazy from the pain, using addiction as escape and a source of dopamine. We grope for anything to soften the pain— to deaden it, to pad it with something—and then we become addicted to whatever it is that seems to do the trick—work, drugs, nicotine, shopping and material consumption, violence, sex, anger, alcohol, caffeine, food, gambling, or internet. All addictions stem from the moment when we met our raw, damaged edge and we simply couldn't stand it. This often evolves into a constellation of addictions, because the first one loses its effectiveness and we'll add in another and another. Running, running, harder and harder, from the soft, raw core of our buried pain.

We've all got trauma. The variations are vast and center around our psychological makeup and questions of extremity. How were you hurt? How often? By what or whom? How long ago? These layers of influence and detail combine into our particular version of messy personhood and life situation. Unfortunately, these important questions aren't typically asked of trauma survivors when bad behavior erupts, nor are the survivors encouraged to heal.

Meanwhile, our news culture tells us about the behavior of a trauma survivor, not their background. Culturally, we focus solely on behavior, wanting to fix or stop bad behavior instead of asking questions about the seed of trauma that grows into the bad behavior. As we discussed earlier, trauma and addiction are culturally met with shame and blame. And so we continue the cycle of suffering.

Whether or not to introduce trauma was a big question for me in writing this book; however, I couldn't exclude such a pivotal contributor to our suffering—to our inability to holistically heal—that I come across daily in my work. Self-worth, and other facets of our health and wholeness, is significantly hobbled by trauma. Unresolved trauma stands, as a forbidding nightclub bouncer might, with arms squarely crossed in the doorway that opens to healing. How on earth could I not include this widely shared experience of mind? Yet this short discussion seems to do trauma a disservice. I'm hopeful that you'll forgive me, and that you'll maybe find a thread from this section that you can follow to the heart of healing. Trauma is a Very Big Topic that may be a good one to explore further, and the Barthel book I mentioned is a good place to start, along with the works of Peter Levine, Gabor Maté, and Byron Katie.

Trauma work is often most helpful when the person seeking to heal is supported by an expert. It's important to note that trauma-induced Energy is stored with pain, which means it's going to release with that pain, and it can be an intense and unpleasant experience. Along with expert help, reading books and participating in group work can be helpful—healing is often aided when we go into our pain so deeply that we see it is not just our pain, but everyone's pain. It's immensely moving and supportive to discover that our pain is not private to us. We may still have addictions of all kinds, but we cease to believe in them as a gateway to happiness. We can start to release some of our shame as we cultivate self-compassion and realize that we're not alone.

That's all to say that there is no easy fix-it for trauma, but you can indeed rewire the past through the present. It's amazing what we can do with curiosity, even in the most incongruent spaces of messy personhood. If we can cultivate curiosity in the middle of chaos, this curiosity changes our perception of the chaos—there's a softening, even if it's ever-so-subtle. The solution to trauma is philosophically simple: compassionately holding space for self or other. **Holding space** is being with a person while consciously embodying awareness, presence, nonjudgment, and love. We offer these feelings of good will while protecting a shared space of acceptance, safety, and comfort. We'll talk more about compassion in the next chapter, but know this: hurt people hurt people; healed people heal people. We must remember that we're not entitled to anything; we can't expect others to meet our needs, because they most often won't. Our only hope in breaking the cycle of trauma is healing our minds. The cultural movement toward the open discussion of trauma—of addressing trauma with the intention of healing—has begun, and it must be supported and fostered. A challenging path. The rewards, however, are considerable, and include peace of mind, compassion, connection, and an open heart. These Ten Healing Practices can help you on the path.

The Ten Healing Practices

There can only be more peace, collaboration, and integration in the world if the world contains more peaceful, collaborative, and integrated people. By fostering our personal evolution—in tending our mind through a more constructive relationship with emotions, stress, and trauma—we contribute to healing on a global scale. There's no tactic, place, person, or policy that can deliver us to well-being, outside of our mind. It must start at the micro (each person), which then instructs the macro (the world); it starts with you, with me, with each of us. Everything we want is denied or granted through the complex power of mind: mind the bridge, or mind the barrier.

We've considered some Very Big topics together—the myths of our culture that keep us stuck, habits, personal responsibility, self-worth, self-care, honoring our body, and tending our mind—and it's possible that, at this point, you're feeling some mixture of intrigue and overwhelm. If mind is the bridge or barrier to all that we desire, then creating more clarity, focus, and equanimity in the mind will support all that we've covered thus far plus everything we'll uncover in the remainder of our exploration together.

Before we begin using the Ten Healing Practices, we must create space—space in our life, space in our schedule, and space in our minds. When we're continually tuned in to the noise of the world and rushing around, we lose connection with ourselves and with the parts of mind that can support us. Maybe our creation of space could involve connecting with nature or simply sitting with a cup of tea and some quiet. Maybe it starts with some breathing snacks or a one-hour-daily technology fast. There are many big and little ways to give ourselves the space that we desperately need in our quest for wholeness. As we give ourselves more space, we gain more clarity and feel more connected to our true selves. Space is healing, on its own.

The Ten Healing Practices support your movement toward more JOY. The information provided for each practice is backed by years of research, experience, and practice, from a scientific and spiritual perspective. Of all of the many, many practices that I've researched and vetted, these ten are the biggest game-changers. The best part about these life-changing practices?

You already know them. There's nothing new to learn because each practice is something that we do naturally when we're in a balanced state. Because what we focus on expands, purposefully exploring these innate tendencies and turning them into practices supports us in creating clarity, equanimity, and focus in the mind.

Splendid.

The Ten Healing Practices are not ordered steps or items on a to-do list that we can check off and voilà, there's our Mind-as-Bridge, complete. They are a journey, a practice, that grows in manifestation over time. Practices are, well, they're things that we practice at. As you and I explore the Ten Healing Practices together, I'll provide a basic explanation of the practice and why it's helpful; an example of how leaning into that practice might help us tend our mind in the trenches of our everyday life; and one or two simple starting practice ideas. I invite you to give each of these practices your full attention, to play with them, and to bring your awareness and curiosity to what transpires in your mind and your life experience over time, as you lean into them in your daily life. The *great news* is that each practice tends to enhance the ease and growth of the others. We'll start with a practice that you're already familiar with.

1. MINDFULNESS: *I NOTICE THAT* . . .

We defined mindfulness as one of the Three Amigos. You've likely also noticed my frequent use of the word. Why is mindfulness such a key practice? Increasing our everyday mindfulness helps us live, heal, intentionally evolve, and supports the other nine practices over time. Mindfulness is a word we hear more and more in mainstream culture now, but my experience is that many people are still confused about what mindfulness is. Alternatively, people are turned off by it because it sounds woo-woo. I can assure you there's nothing woo-woo about mindfulness.

Mindfulness is attention to the present moment in its fullness, without judgment. This sounds fairly ordinary, but it's in direct opposition to the manner in which many of us navigate our days. Mindfulness is being aware of the fullness of now—connected to who we are, what we're doing, and what we're experiencing—while quieting judgment of, and resistance to, what *is*. Mindfulness begins with the body, where we take the time to pay attention to our physical body interacting with our environment. We then expand that focus to keen awareness of what's happening right now—physical sensations, emotions, thoughts—minus our opinion of it. Mindfulness is meditation in action. At its best, mindfulness becomes a way of life, reducing stress and emotional drama and increasing the joy of the present moment.

With mindfulness, we're more likely to view a challenging moment as simply that—a challenging moment—instead of an experience that's ruined our whole day/week/year/life. We're more likely to see people's flaws as simple flaws rather than traits that paint them entirely in one color.

Mindfulness supports us in purposefully taking a mental step back in order to notice what's happening, and helps us to avoid immediately engaging with intense emotions and reactions. Mindfulness isn't a judge. It's more akin to a doting older sister looking after her younger one in an alert and caring way. It's an optimal interaction between our attention and our environment, including the people around us.

Here is an example of how our lack of mindfulness makes our life less joyful: If I'm walking down a crowded city sidewalk on my way to a job interview, I need to be present. But if I'm absorbed in thinking about the argument I just had with the manager of my child's daycare center, I'm setting myself up for what I call "the debacles of distraction." Contrary to popular belief, our mind can only truly focus on one thing at a time; our multitasking ability, though much glamorized, is an illusion. So if I'm walking along, thinking about the argument and rehashing it in my mind, I'm feeding the fire of my own anger. That anger would distort my perception and feelings. I'd be so lost in thought that I wouldn't be aware of anything else around me—the ever-so-slight pressure on my backpack of someone slipping my wallet out, or storm clouds gathering in the sky above me, about to dump copious amounts of rain on my umbrella-less self, minutes before my job interview.

When we're wrapped up in our thoughts, we miss a lot. In this scenario, my lack of mindfulness would affect my focus and composure during the job interview. For starters, I'd be in a bad mood, have no ID, and be wet.

If instead I chose to put the conversation with the daycare manager aside and focus on the matter at hand—walking my commute and noticing sights, sounds, people, terrain, sky, as well as my body moving through all that— things might unfold quite differently. Mindfulness in the moment would have served my ultimate goals, as I would likely have arrived to the interview dry, focused, and able to validate my identity. I also would likely have enjoyed my commute more. When we lack mindfulness in our daily life, the same thing happens. We become wrapped up in our thoughts and emotions about the past or future, losing sight of the bigger picture. Our perspective narrows, and we lose our way. We do and say things that cause suffering, for ourselves and others. Mindfulness creates a space of full engagement with the moment, where we can more clearly see our options, be aware of positive things to move toward (an umbrella purchase), and notice negative things to move away from (a pickpocket).

Mindfulness also creates powerful positive change in our inner landscape. One way I'll mention here is that it gives us the power to change our past conditioning. When we're listening and responding mindfully, with our focus on the present moment, we notice our thoughts more; we notice more about body language, intention, triggers, and habitual thinking in how we relate to others. When we're practicing mindfulness, we have a better chance of rewiring the neural circuitry that produces the unquestioned thoughts, beliefs, and behaviors that trip us up each day. We start practicing mindfulness by simply noticing the present moment, in its fullness.

Simple Starting Practice: Daily Doses of Mindfulness

Each day, choose one simple physical task—washing dishes, bathing your baby, drinking tea, taking a shower, filling your bag lunch with Food Sass—and practice mindfulness. This means fully experiencing what you're doing with the attention of a six-month-old, and gently bringing your mind back when it wanders to past or future (which it will). For instance, when washing dishes, you can notice how easily the water comes from the spout and how warm it feels on your hands. You can watch as your hands do the job seemingly all on their own. You might enjoy how well the soap works with its soft, crazy bubbles, and how fragrant it smells. Maybe you notice the sound of the sponge on the dish as it gets squeaky clean, or maybe you notice that feeling of satisfaction you get from clearing the sink. The focus is to simply do dishes and notice all that you take in with your five senses as part of the dish-doing process, along with what pops up in your mind, recognizing what you need to gently let go (which is everything unless it has to do with the dish you're washing right now).

2. GRATITUDE: *I AM THANKFUL FOR* . . .

Gratitude is the gateway drug to inner peace. For most folks, it's the simplest and most accessible of these ten practices. **Gratitude** is being thankful for what feels good to us in our life experience. I can mindfully connect to gratitude for so many things in my life, big and small: my two able legs; the lilac-smelling breeze coming in the open window while I write; a home; birdsong; work that I love; creativity; the earthy smell of woods after rain; true-blue friends; my family; and a heart that pumps faithfully approximately 100,000 times a day, independent of my conscious bidding. Once we start feeling grateful, we sometimes notice there's no end of things to recognize with gratitude: the way our magnificent body breathes for us; clean water; how plankton and plants work together to make oxygen to support animal life; the joy of a kick-ass vacation experience; and the feeling of warm sunshine on our skin.

The practice of gratitude isn't about feeling happy, happy, happy all the time. That's a lot to ask of any practice. Life can feel hard at times, and sometimes we simply feel miserable and ungrateful and that's all fine. Still, through an intentional gratitude practice, we can begin to feel grateful and abundant a little more regularly. We start to appreciate more and more of our life experience in whatever form that life experience takes. This leads to increased joy, and focusing on what we're grateful for can turn our focus toward our abundance and away from feelings of lack. This state, however often we can bring ourselves there, has powerful healing powers. It feels good, which is certainly a bonus; *and* the vibration of gratitude and abundance affects each cell in your body and everything around you.

Simple Starting Practice 1: Keep a Gratitude Journal

A gratitude journal is a game-changer. If you stick to it on the majority of days, you'll feel a positive shift in the way you feel about your life. Start by gifting yourself with something to log your gratitude in. It can be as simple as a spiral notebook with lined paper or it can be a lovely brown leather-bound journal with a gold-embossed cover. If you're someone who wants to type gratitude into your smartphone or computer, that works too. However, I'd still urge you to try an analog approach, as the physical pen-to-paper writing is important for many of us.

Physical pen-to-paper writing has extra power in that writing helps us connect our mind and body. It also combines our gratitude practice with a mini technology fast, which can be helpful for building the dedicated space for our gratitude to bloom and grow. That space can be hard to hold if you're distracted by incoming tweets or texts.

A gratitude practice is simple and powerful. Each day, preferably at around the same time, sit and create a list of things that you're thankful for. It helps to include big and small things, tangible and intangible things, and to have a minimum of five. Why the minimum? There will be days when you sit down with some *serious* gratitude attitude. During those times when life seems terrible or when everything seems to be going wrong, it's hard to imagine feeling grateful for a-n-y-thing. This is the time that we need this practice most as it brings some much-needed perspective to our mind. Coming up with five things for my gratitude journal has saved my sanity on many dark-feeling days. This practice is transformative, in the moment and cumulatively increasing joy over time.

I recommended a lovely brown leather-bound writing journal with a gold-embossed cover earlier because it was the choice of a recent student. She requested it as a birthday gift from her daughter after my event, because she felt that, given her just-getting-by financial situation and resulting feelings of lack, writing in this journal would feel luxurious for her. This journal gives her pleasure each day, and brings a feeling of material abundance to a small corner of her life. I like writing in a spiral-bound notebook with colored markers. Choose what feels good to write in, for you, and journal your gratitude.

Simple Starting Practice 2: Saying Thanks

Each night at dinner, have each person take a turn saying a minimum of two things that they're grateful for out loud. My family calls this ritual Saying Thanks. We started this practice when my sons were young, and we say thanks whether there's two of us or six of us, whether it's our family alone, or whether guests are present. I tell our guests that this is our gratitude practice, and they're welcome to join or not, with no judgment. I've been amazed over the years, as my sons grew up, that their friends who were over for dinner would almost always choose to join in on Saying Thanks, often wanting to go first. The two rules that most folks find helpful are 1) You have to say at least two things you're grateful for; and 2) They can't be covertly negative, such as, "I'm thankful that my brother is an idiot." Yes, that's a real-life example that one of my sons came up with one night, hence the creation of rule number two. You definitely don't need to be eating with a family to do this—you can also order up a gratitude meal routine for one.

3. HUMOR: *I CAN LAUGH AT . . .*

Laughter is fun and feels good, and it's good for us. It relieves stress and opens our hearts. It connects us to others from a place of lightheartedness. Laughter reminds us that life is a gift, deflating something that might have seemed like a huge, hairy deal only moments ago into a medium, relatively hairless deal. Laughter unequivocally underscores that joy can be ours. Humor can be a ray of sunshine, breaking through the dark cloud of the troubles that weigh us down.

So, call your funniest friend. Watch videos or read books that make you laugh. No matter how many times I read *Sh*t My Dad Says* by Justin Halpern, there are sections that make me giggle every time. Seek out time with people who like to have *fun* and enjoy some lighthearted play. We're looking for funny that simply *is*. Jim Carrey and Dick Van Dyke, for me, in their endless array of facial and body expressions, are just funny, even if they say nothing. One of my clients watches bird videos and cat videos on YouTube for laughter. Calvin and Hobbes cartoons make me laugh. In addition to Bill Watterson being a comic genius, I find the mind of boys fun and funny.

We can also invoke the healing power of laughter via voluntary laughter—called laughter yoga—where we laugh for no reason at all. Similar to all of these practices, humor is self-expansive, meaning it feeds on itself and feeds all of the other healing practices as well.

What tickles your funny bone?

Simple Starting Practice: Find a Laughter Go-To

Look back through recent years and come up with one book, movie, podcast series, joke, cartoon, sitcom episode, or video theme that tends to make you chuckle. Pull it out several times a week, especially when things are feeling hard or bleak. This practice isn't about putting your head in the sand; it's about allowing humor to lighten our perspective and open our heart a bit. Find one you particularly enjoy? Share it, in person, with a friend or colleague and relish in the delight of shared laughter. Shared laughter is connective and healing.

4. SIMPLICITY: *I AM NOT DEFINED BY* . . .

Antoine de Saint-Exupéry wrote, "Perfection is achieved not when there is nothing more to add, but when there is nothing left to take away." How true. Often, less is truly more. Each thing that we own, each responsibility we take on, comes packaged with mental clutter, duties, and maintenance needs. I'm not suggesting that we need to go live alone in a mountaintop yurt, but selectively simplifying is freeing and naturally moves us closer to Ourselves.

We need to be especially mindful of material things that we feel define us. This attachment to the material status symbols of life can weigh us down and has the potential to warp our sense of who we are. In Western cultures, we spend an awful lot of our time, energy, and money on accumulation. The Japanese poet Ryōkan Taigu was right when he wrote, "If you want to find the meaning, stop chasing after so many things."

Simple Starting Practice: Declutter

Set yourself a realistic goal to start getting rid of stuff that takes up space in your home and your life and isn't serving you. For example, each month, you might fill one box with things you don't need anymore and get rid of it via Big Brothers Big Sisters pick-up, Salvation Army, Freecycle, Craigslist, eBay, or the garbage. It's amazing how freeing it feels to remove a little clutter and complexity and breathe some space into our lives. This can also extend to how we spend our time. You might periodically review your schedule to uncover if there are roles, jobs, or tasks in your life that can be softened or released. There are many ways to create more simplicity in our lives. Start small and steady and see how it feels.

5. GENEROSITY: *I CAN GIVE . . .*

When we're intentionally generous, it not only brings happiness to others, it brings joy to us as well. There are many forms of generosity—for me, the most meaningful generosities are those of time, heart, and spirit.

Generosity of time is when we contribute our time to support another's well-being, most especially when we're mindfully present during that time. A few years back, shortly after my divorce, I got body-slammed by pneumonia. I was flat on my back for over a week. Several friends—all with full and busy lives—delivered groceries, shoveled my walkway, made me soup, and came by to check on me. These generosities of time meant the world to me. Yes, these acts kept me shoveled and fed and breathing the healing smell of chicken soup; they also helped me feel supported during a vulnerable time and guarded me from feeling isolated when I was sick.

Generosity of heart is when we assume the best in others. For example, when someone lets us down, we choose generous thoughts to explain it. Instead of thinking that my friend didn't call me back because he's unreliable and rude, I can choose a more generous thought such as, *"I hope everything's okay with him,"* or, *"Maybe he didn't get my message."* I may find out that he *was* being unreliable and rude, but even in that case, leading with generous thoughts brings me peace in the meantime.

Generosity of spirit is a tough one to explain, but we know it when it's offered to us. It's that feeling when someone is fully present for us. It's when we meet eyes with someone, and they *see* us and we *see* them.

Neuroscience has shown that the reward centers in our brain light up as strongly when we give as when we receive, often even more so. Our generosity of time, heart, spirit, money, and thoughtfulness give to us as much as they give to others.

There's a yellow light in expressing generosity: expecting thanks, gratitude, pats on the back, or Facebook likes in return for our generosity. This yellow light, like a cautionary traffic light, helps us pause to see that we're making our generosity about ourselves and our desire for validation. It's no longer generosity, but a sort of validation bribe. Authentic generosity is freely giving of our possessions, time, heart, and/or spirit. As we work with our generosity practice, it's helpful to learn to let go of that anticipated feedback-cookie. One way to work with letting go is to regularly commit generous acts that no one sees you do, and that you tell no one about. Only you know that you gave a homeless woman a blanket or cleaned the snow off your elderly neighbor's car. This helps us lean into what authentic generosity is all about, which is giving of the self out of love and joy.

Simple Starting Practice: Offer Generosity

Take a page out of Winston Churchill's book. He said, "We make a living by what we get, but we make a life by what we give." Look for places where you can offer your generosity. Take the time to notice how this changes the receiver and how it changes you. Even something simple such as inviting the person carrying only three items behind you in the grocery checkout line to go ahead of you creates an Energetic shift in both parties, and often in the cashier, as well. Our amigo of awareness can help us in our generosity practice. As we notice our environment more, we bring attention to areas where we can be generous with our time, resources, and spirit.

6. PERSPECTIVE: *I CHOOSE TO SEE* . . .

Our **perspective** is how we see or interpret the world around us. Perspective is often instructed by our habitual assumptions—our ideas about How Things Are—which often keep us from seeing anything in a fresh, open way. The first step in turning perspective into a healing practice is to remember that our perspective is simply that—*our perspective.* Our thoughts, our opinions, our factual-feeling assertions, are only one tiny representation of what's possible. We must remember that our take on something is only one take, and that there are 7.6 billion people in this wild, beautiful world who each have a unique perspective—on everything.

Many influences affect our perspective. Our personality, our intellectual intelligence, our emotional intelligence, our romantic relationships, our gender identity, our parents, our children, our religious and spiritual beliefs, our families, our friends, our age, our environment, our culture, our schoolteachers and coaches, our neighbors, our jobs, our bosses, our financial situation, our employees, our exposure to other cultures, our physical body, our talents, and our challenges all affect our perspective, and that's the short list. Suffice it to say that we each come to the table with a unique way of seeing things.

The practice of bringing awareness to our perspective helps us remember that the very things we complain about and are resentful of have other sides to them, if we only choose to see them. For instance, I sometimes complain about having to drive my teenage sons all over creation. Another perspective is that the time we spend in the car often allows for precious connection and conversation, and I know I'll miss it someday and then wonder what on earth I was complaining about.

An easy way to shift perspective—to reframe a "chore" as a thing to feel grateful for—is to start the sentence with *"I get to"* instead of *"I have to."* Instead of *"I have to drive my kids around,"* I think, *"I get to drive my kids around and talk to them."* Instead of Bill of Bill's Garbage Trucking thinking, *"I have to work when some of my friends are retired,"* he thinks, *"I get to wake up each day and earn money for contributing to pollution control."* Over the years, when I remember to invoke this perspective shift, I've found the phrase *"I get to"* to be uplifting and empowering.

The fact that we each have our perspective makes the world a vastly more intriguing place. A tangible example of this is visual artists like Van Gogh, Monet, and O'Keeffe, who saw the world with unique perspectives and were able to communicate through visual art. The flip side of our ability to have a unique take on the world is that it can be challenging for us to see things any way but our way. I can think of many times when I felt that I was misunderstood due to perspective. I can also think of many times when I was unable or unwilling to see something through another's perspective.

Our perspective is typically habitual, and we have the power to make it a choice. Auschwitz survivor Viktor Frankl taught that our perspective toward life is our singular and most ultimate freedom. However, like most of these practices, the concept is simple, and the practice isn't always easy. But the benefits are profound. Our perspective practice also helps us more easily utilize the other healing practices, such as gratitude, generosity, compassion, humility, and forgiveness.

Simple Starting Practice 1: Circle Back

Next time someone's words or actions annoy you, circle back to the situation later in your mind. When you've circled back, pretend you're trying to defend, to a third party, how and why the other person spoke or acted the way they did. This is akin to a debate class in school, where you're given a side to argue for, which could be something you disagree with, even vehemently. You might have to dig deep to try and see the other side's perspective enough that you can argue to defend it. Doing this in your everyday life can be a helpful reminder to hold space for other people who have a different take on things.

Simple Starting Practice 2: Listen

When you're having a disagreement with another person, simply stop talking and listen. Truly listen. If you still feel angry, hurt, confused, or misunderstood, you might say to them, *"This is really hard for me. I disagree with you, but I also wonder if I'm not understanding you. Please help me understand your perspective on this."* Soften your defenses and let your old amigo, curiosity, guide you.

7. MEDITATION: *I RETURN TO* . . .

A few short decades ago, meditation was little-known here in the West and was classified squarely in the woo-woo department. Today, the Western version of meditation is popular with elite athletes, moms, hedge-fund managers, dads, CEOs, teachers, political leaders, entrepreneurs, college students, scientists, tradespeople, and creatives—a wide array of enthusiasts. Meditation is also being taken more seriously by scientists, as its benefits are more widely recognized and confirmed. Among other things, meditation helps us to improve mental focus; increase creativity and insight; lower stress and improve our stress resilience; increase patience and joy; slow our heart rate; decrease depression and pain; and realize our innate capacity to become a more fully conscious being, beyond our five senses. And nothing helps create a positive, open mindset as quickly and completely as meditation.

Meditation costs no money, takes a modest amount of time, and we can do it anywhere. Meditation trains us in awareness and compassion and helps us to develop perspective. Meditation is related to mindfulness, so you might notice some similarities between the discussion that follows and our previous explorations of mindfulness. Meditation requires mindfulness, and mindfulness is part of meditation. Both serve to discipline and focus mind.

What is meditation? **Meditation** begins with the simple act of focusing our mind on one thing, often the breath, making it both an experience and a skill. The essence of meditation is a heightened state of awareness in this very moment, bringing the mind back to this point of focus, continually and without judgment. We can also try watching thoughts. What quiets is not the thoughts themselves, but our attachment to, and involvement with the thoughts. Meditation trains our mind to pay attention by allowing thoughts to flow naturally—in the way that we might watch leaves float by in a river rather than running into the river and grabbing the leaves to deeply analyze them. When the thoughts arise (and they will), we can simply notice the thoughts, and then quietly and gently label them—without tone or judgment—as *thinking*. We then return to a light and gentle focus on our breath. Not controlling or changing the breath in any way, just keeping our light attention on the sensation of breathing—the rise and fall of our chest, the expansion and contraction of our rib cage, the movement of our belly, and the sensations in our windpipe and at the tip of our nose. And we simply keep doing that. Meditation is simple in concept, but it's most definitely a practice.

Over time, as our practice strengthens, our meditation comes "off the cushion" so to speak. Meaning, the lessons we learn while sitting in meditation start to infuse our daily lives. We notice that our stream of thought has little gaps in it which allow us space from our constant thinking, emoting, and mental machinations. Meditation leads to less judgment, toward self and other, as we start to see that our labeling things good or bad is simply thinking. You see, meditation isn't about becoming metaphysically complicated but is instead about appreciating simplicity. As we get the hang of neither indulging nor repressing our thoughts—of how it feels to simply notice—we sow the seeds of becoming more content and joyful in the midst of our daily lives in a wild world. This is huge.

Some folks find a meditation definition like this to be a bit abstract or esoteric. Meditation is one of those things that we need to try out for a bit in order to understand it, kind of like learning how to ride a bike, which can sound confusing and weird when someone tries to explain it to us. Similar to several topics that we've been curious about together, understanding what meditation *is* can be helped by understanding what it's *not*.

Meditation is not a nap or a vacation from irritation. It's not a drifting off somewhere or daydreaming or in any way moving away from yourself. On the contrary, it's a return to yourself. We're not checking *out* during meditation, we're checking *in*. Although meditation has a rich history in some religions and philosophies, meditation is for anyone, regardless of their belief in a higher power and regardless of their religious affiliation. A final common misconception is that meditation is about emptying the mind, and I can assure you that pursuing a goal of emptying the mind or of stopping thoughts is a one-way ticket to frustration, which is the opposite of meditation's intent. This is a good time to flesh out the intent of meditation.

I alluded to a "Western version" of meditation earlier. You may have wondered, *"Huh? There's versions of meditation?"* Yes, there are. Meditation, as it's been used in the East for millennia, has the goal of connecting to the higher self—to spirit—and of becoming a way of living one's life. Some Eastern meditation traditions note several stages, such as concentration, meditation, contemplation, illumination, and inspiration. In the East, the stage that is recognized to engross the meditator for many, many years is *concentration*. The intention of this stage of Eastern meditation is learning to focus the mind and to use it in its focused state. This first stage is what we typically call *meditation* in the West, and it's what we've been discussing here. We also discussed physical, emotional, and mental benefits, and this alone is what some folks are looking to get out of the Western version of meditation.

Many others are looking to meditation as a way to connect with a higher power—the God of their understanding. Meditation, similar to prayer or chanting, is an act that can move us into a personal relationship with a higher power. We won't find the God of our understanding in our intellect. Divine communion happens from our spirit aspect, and quieting and focusing our mind activates our bridging mind (as opposed to our barrier mind). We may also notice that the honesty, kindness, and humor that we show ourselves as we attempt to quiet our mind are far more inspiring and helpful than any kind of religious or spiritual striving, for or against anything. Meditation has the power to open all of that snazziness up, if that's our intention. Regardless of the intention, meditation is a healing practice in so many ways, and neuroscience studies have even shown that it physically and chemically changes our brain for the better.

I spent extra time in introducing you to this practice of meditation because it's powerful, but getting started can feel intimidating or frustrating. You *will* become irritated. You may sometimes feel like a meditation failure. You will absolutely have periods of being restless, fidgety, annoyed, angry, bored, etc. That's all normal, and you're just a person; please don't be hard on yourself. The key is to simply notice any of that and watch it. All of those things tend to quiet if we watch them and name them instead of trying to resist them or pretend they're not happening.

Simple Starting Practice: Schedule Consistent Practice

The most important thing in creating a meditation practice is consistency. Find a time each day to commit to five minutes of meditation in your schedule, and do this for about a month. Over time you can choose to increase to ten to fifteen minutes (or longer), but this is not a race, and there's no achievement or awards ceremony. It's not a contest for how long you sit there; it's a practice in gradually lengthening your ability to focus and concentrate—meditation trains the mind. If you're eager for more instruction, a clear and well-constructed website is Headspace; they also have a snazzy app that you can use to support your meditation practice—free to start and then paid. There are 100 percent free apps as well, like Insight Timer. My personal favorite online meditation support is *The Practice of Living Awareness*; it's *free* online meditation training through Spirit Fire Retreat Center. It's a rich mindfulness meditation practice with time-tested steps and structure that lead the participant on a journey over fourteen weeks. I highly recommend it.

8. HUMILITY: *I FOCUS OUTWARDLY ON . . .*

Humility, and the related word *humble,* is connected to a practice that helps to broaden our heart, our mind, and our ability to demonstrate compassion. It's also a subtle practice with some imitations that are inauthentic. Let's start with what humility isn't. Being humble does not mean, as some imagine (and as some dictionaries describe), "having a low opinion of oneself." That, Mr. Dictionary, is called low self-worth.

The meaning of "being humbled" has been distorted in present-day mainstream politics, sports, business, and self-marketing to become a catch-phrase vehicle for boasting about things that make us look good. This is imitation humility, which is closely related to false modesty. I recently saw a marketing email from an online motivation guy that said, "Hey, my Facebook followers just topped 1.2 million and I am just so humbled by you guys." This is not humility. This is self-aggrandizement and conceit. I'm not raining on his Facebook follower parade; I'm simply pointing out that this is not "being humbled." Instead, it's a *humblebrag* that uses the word *humble* as a smoke-screen to brag about our expertise, our achievements, our prowess.

The opposite of humility is conceit; conceit is an ingenious creature, at times hiding behind masks of humility, empathy, or virtue. We see the word *humbled* misused when athletes are "humbled" by winning the championship; a social-media star is "humbled" by the outpouring of attention from her fans; a politician is "humbled" by being appointed to a position of power; or charity volunteers are "humbled" by the recognition of their public efforts. These examples are not humility, and a humble person would not likely call themselves humble or humbled. As Martin Luther wrote, "True humility does not know that it is humble. If it did, it would be proud from the contemplation of so fine a virtue."

Instead, a humble person most often doesn't call themselves anything because they don't think about themselves much at all; and when they do, they don't imagine themselves as being more or less than others. They simply are. **Humility** is a tendency to focus outward. Humble folks have a real interest in others and in the world at large. They tend to operate from a base of compassion, generosity, gratitude, and kindness—many of the practices that we're talking about in the Ten Healing Practices. Around 500 BC, Confucius defined humility as "the solid foundation of all virtues." While humility is often associated with nonassertiveness, passivity, and meekness, as noted earlier, true humility is incredibly powerful. Examples of well-known folks who consistently demonstrate(d) humility are Abraham Lincoln, Jane Goodall, Mother Teresa, and the 14th Dalai Lama. Humble folks like these keep their accomplishments, gifts, and talents in proper perspective and, again, don't think about themselves much in the first place. A humble person tends to be self-aware, and has a dispassionate awareness of their limitations, as a unique individual and as a human.

We can be put in direct touch with our humility when faced by humiliation, failure, being wrong, or some other perceived calamity. We receive lessons in humility when we think we're some special and infallible superhuman, and then come face-to-face with evidence to the contrary. We can also feel humility in relation to something so immense, grand, or meaningful—history, nature, felt connection to the God of our understanding—that our personal insignificance becomes palpable.

Simple Starting Practice: Reflect and Share Your Humanity

When you find yourself putting yourself above or below someone else or a group of someone elses, notice it and give yourself time to reflect on your shared humanity and all of the things that you have in common with the others. Some other avenues toward humility you can take are to listen more than you talk, admit when you're wrong, and remember that almost anything you say could be wrong. Spend time in nature and around children—their beauty and power will surely kindle humility. Finally, the healing practice of gratitude naturally generates humility.

9. FORGIVENESS: *I RELEASE FEELINGS OF . . .*

There's no one who's unforgivable. There's also no one who's incapable of forgiving. Contrary to the saying "Forgive and forget," forgiveness doesn't mean that we forget what someone has said or done. It doesn't mean we say to our cheating spouse upon finding them in our bed with a lover, *"Oh, I know you have a messy personhood just like all of us, and therefore you are forgiven for lying to me and dishonoring our monogamous bond. Tomorrow's a new day."* It *could* be that, if we're a free spirit who has no attachment to fidelity in marriage. Historically, though, infidelity is a tough one for the majority of people, hence my example. Emotional turbulence, as we've discussed, can be powerful and challenging, and it can bring out the worst in us.

The path to forgiveness doesn't include shame and blame; nor does it involve harm, meanness, violence, or suppressing our truth. What, exactly, does the path to forgiveness look like? Recall that emotional pain requires us to move through it; moving through emotional pain and grievances is not a one-time act or statement. Real forgiveness is rarely a Hallmark card moment, with hugs and tears of forgiveness. More often, it's a messy, loud, thrashing-about process with some of that two-steps-forward, one-step-back action. **Forgiveness** is an ongoing, conscious decision made by our whole selves to release our feelings of resentment or vengeance. We decide that we want to choose healing over external vengeance—that we'll take the longer, more difficult path of what's right, instead of the shorter path of what's easy. Take heart, because the truth about forgiveness is that it heals the person who does the hard work of forgiveness even more than it heals those who have intentionally or unintentionally challenged our emotions.

Without forgiveness, we remain shackled to the person who we believe harmed us. And until we forgive that person, they hold the keys to our freedom. We must flex our personal responsibility muscles and take ownership of our emotions and outcomes. Forgiveness is the only way to release the past, heal, and live fully in the present.

"This sounds weird. So, the insulting things that my father-in-law said at my wife's fiftieth birthday party—you're saying that I own that?"

Not at all. We can never own anything about another person. I'm saying you own 100 percent of the way *you feel*, 100 percent of what you said, and 100 percent of what you did. Why 100 percent? For most of us, the power of forgiveness arises from the balance point of a triangle: we acknowledge the other person's humanity—that they are messy and imperfect like us; we own our words, emotions, and actions; and we respond to the other person's words and behavior that *we feel* were wrong, with clarity and firmness. Ideally, the other person's job is to also own their contributions to the problem.

Remember, however, that the real problem is *our* resentment, so the other person may have no idea they breached our boundaries. When we focus on our circle of influence around resentment, we realize that there are only three items that live in that circle: *our* words, *our* actions, and *our* emotions. Emotions commonly involved in resentment are disgust, disappointment, hurt, embarrassment, sadness, anger, and blame. A motley crew indeed. Blame, in particular, causes much pain for all parties involved. Moreover, if we're trying to split up blame— *"Well, I'll own 35 percent of what went down. I acted a bit badly, but it was because my father-in-law did x, y, and z that I acted badly at all"*—it's impossible to release and forgive. We're hanging on, squabbling in our little mind about who was the bigger jerk, and our mind almost always gives the other person the Biggest Jerk Award. Does it matter?

I know this 35 percent gig intimately. It can be a difficult thing to look in the mirror and say, *"The buck stops here. I own all of these shitty feelings that I'm having."* I can tell you that when we start to bring forgiveness into our relationships with others, and our relationship with ourselves, the world this process opens up is often not-so-pretty. It can feel easier and more comfortable to be self-righteous and assume that it was all the other person's fault, that our bad behavior is because of them, which is not the case. This is another school-of-life situation, when it's best not to focus on the result but instead to focus on the process.

Forgiveness, like grief, is not an event or an emotion. It's a journey, a process that happens over time as we put down the baggage of our resentment and grievances, moment by moment. Curiosity, awareness, and self-honesty often help us to see, over time, that we also played a part in the grievance. We can choose to keep ourselves in bondage by dragging around all we haven't forgiven of others, and ourselves, in the past, or we can choose not to. In many ways, we forgive out of self-interest: *I forgive because I want out of my pain.* We're not held back by the love and good behavior that we didn't receive in the past, but by the love and good behavior that we're not extending in the present. Remember, I'm not saying this is easy, but I *am* saying it's worth it.

A two-for-one deal is that when we forgive, we release critical judgment of ourselves as well as others. We lighten up. We don't cling to negative experiences that result from decisions that we made while learning in the School of Life. We don't define ourselves by them. That's regret. Regret is an invisible weight on our back, which can get heavier as the years go by and our grievances accumulate. Self-forgiveness is imperative to healing, BodyMindSpirit. Zen teacher Charlotte Joko-Beck wrote in *Nothing Special: Living Zen*, "I will forgive even if it takes me a lifetime of practice . . . because the quality of our whole life is on the line." Beyond the self, the practice of forgiveness has the power to create the peaceful planet that we all desire. This is not an easy path. Like most things, forgiveness most often happens in layers over time. At a certain point, we forgive because we decide to forgive. Because we have a deep longing to restore balance and wholeness to ourselves, to our relationships, and to our species.

Simple Starting Practice: Find the Lessons

When you find yourself struggling with a grievance, remind yourself that forgiveness can be hard, and that there's no imposed timeline. List some things that you enjoy or admire about the person who you feel has wronged you, or note an important lesson that you learned from what went down. This act helps to bring us out of polarity and blame and start turning our wheels in a different direction or perspective—even if it's a slight shift—about our thoughts and feelings about the other person. This can be an especially freeing practice if the person we haven't forgiven is ourselves.

10. THE PRESENT: *I APPRECIATE NOW BECAUSE* . . .

I appreciate that right now is called **the present**, because it's truly a gift. The present moment is our delicious dance partner, our wondrous lover, and our unwavering constant companion. We often miss out on the present, which is interesting because it's the only thing that's real, in each moment of our lives. We waste our mental capacity and create inner conflict because we're worried about the past (which can lead to stress and depression) or worried about the future (which can lead to stress and anxiety). We can't change the past; we can only learn from it. We can't know or control the future; we can only set intentions and move toward them. The real questions are: *"What's happening now?"*—and then a moment later—*"How about now?"* Our life experience becomes immeasurably less stressful, and more enjoyable, by fully inhabiting the present moment. This sounds lovely, and seems simple, but can be quite challenging.

I learned this lesson when I was twenty-six years old and in the middle of a six-year dental-health saga. At that point, I had an appointment with an oral surgeon in Boston to have him remove the roots of one of my molars to see if that root was causing an ongoing infection. I liked this guy. He was a straight shooter who had a very real and shoulder-to-shoulder approach in his patient interactions.

The procedure started with local anesthetic, which was then followed by him going into the small space of my mouth with his big hands and cutting up my gums and tooth. I was terrified. I was terrified in a general way from dental PTSD. This was the third major procedure on this poor tooth, and I had the growing feeling that all the dental professionals I had seen were shooting in the dark and hoping to hit upon a solution. I was also terrified in a specific way because, similar to a lot of people, I'm not a fan of needles or of someone cutting into my flesh. What if the anesthetic didn't work? Would I feel him slicing through my sensitive gum tissue? Was the little mini-saw that he was going to use on the roots of my tooth loud? What if he slipped? Did he get a good night's sleep the night before?

This cloud of panicked thought is what our untrained mind sounds like a lot of the time. We're neurologically wired, through millions of years of evolution, to suss out where things might go wrong. These thoughts originate in the part of our brain called the *reticular activating system,* or *RAS.* This sussing-out in our RAS is helpful if we're a caveman out on a hunt for a huge woolly mammoth that could squash us like a bug, or impale us like a marshmallow with one of her long tusks. It's less helpful if we're lying on a reclining chair in the oral surgeon's air conditioned office with Mozart playing. One is a relatively controlled situation where we've intentionally handed a complicated job over to a highly trained professional, the other is . . . well, it's not.

The surgeon noticed I was nervous. He stopped what he was doing, put everything down, and looked at me. He said, "Listen, I work on athletes from the Patriots, the Celtics, the Bruins, and the Sox, and I can't tell you how often these guys are shaking in their boots—sometimes crying—as they sit in this chair. You're not alone in your apprehension. I have some advice for you and it's the exact same advice I give to a 350-pound offensive lineman who sits in this chair, freaking out. Focus on exactly what's happening. Don't think about what might happen or what could happen. Just focus on your actual experience in the moment."

He wasn't being esoteric; he was simply pointing out that what I'm experiencing now is the only thing that *is*. The rest is just conjecture and has the unwanted side effect of triggering my fight-or-flight system. I was not going to fight the oral surgeon, nor was I going to flee from him. The remainder of the appointment went much better. Each time my thinking moved to drama and storytelling about what might happen, I brought my mind back to what was presently happening in my mouth. Sometimes, when my untrained mind got on a roll, and he sensed me tensing, he'd calmly repeat, "Remember to focus on exactly what's happening, right now," as he continued working.

My perspective shifted a bit that day. Up to that point, it had never occurred to me to question what my mind was running off with. The idea that I had some influence over the focus of my thoughts was new to me. I'd never realized how much of my emotional misery was about things that might never happen. That the present is a gift.

Now, as awesome as all that is, I can tell you that no matter how much we've read, studied, or experienced, mindfully living in the present isn't an easy adjustment to make. We keep at it by holding the space of gently focused presence as often as possible, experiencing the now. We're not trying to understand, change, fix, or otherwise impact anything. We're simply present with what is. If these ideas sounds vaguely familiar, it's no coincidence that *mindfulness* and *the present* are the bookends of the Ten Healing Practices. Mindfulness leads to more consistent living in the present.

Living in the present increases our mindfulness. We become ever-more fully present to the only reality, which is now.

Simple Starting Practice: Come Back to This Moment

Next time you start to feel anxious or stressed, create a space. Notice. How are things for you right now? Invite yourself to be exquisitely present in this moment. Keep bringing your mind back to right now.

For example, let's say you're riding the subway to work and it's crowded and slow, and it's looking as if you're going to be late for your meeting. First, if there's an action to take, take it. Maybe you can contact someone, if that's possible and appropriate, and tell them you're running late. And then put your timepiece (phone, watch, grandfather clock) away. It makes no sense to keep checking the time to see how late you are, because you'll get there as fast as you get there. Checking the time will only make you feel worse. Now, mindfully focus on your environment and your passing feelings and thoughts. Notice the way the subway car slightly sways. If you're sitting, notice how it feels against your butt and back. Notice the people around you, one by one. Is there someone who needs your seat more than you? (An opportunity to express generosity!) Notice your shoulders. Are they up high around your ears? Allow them to drop naturally down and back. Notice your stomach. Is it tight and ready for battle? Soften it, and breathe from your diaphragm.

Next thing you know, you'll be walking to your meeting from the subway stop, and you'll be as late as you'll be. In the meantime, you've stayed present to your experience. Your heart rate and hormone levels would have stayed normal, helping you avert the health-eroding effects of psychological stress. You wouldn't have generated pit stains on your snazzy shirt and you would show up to the meeting feeling composed. Later, you could review what you might have done differently to be on time. This is an important point.

Being fully in the present doesn't mean that we la-dee-da through life, not planning or running damage control after things go wrong. It means that in the moment, you choose to focus on your circle of influence and not get your undies in a bunch about your circle of concern. As always, I encourage you to be honest, kind, and gentle with yourself while giving your attention to the present. Rinse and repeat.

Tend Your Mind

Our typical pursuit of health, joy, and personal evolution finds us spending immense effort, time, and money trying to get something outside of ourselves to be different—events, circumstances, people, conversations—when what we need is right inside of us, which is the ability to tend our mind. As we tend our mind, there's a softening. A blurring of the lines separating black from white, a shift in our view of self and other, a widening of our perspective, and a gentle attention to what's sometimes called our inner life. In our inner life, opinions become questions and it becomes hard to pick a side. There, we see that changing the world is about changing our minds. We see that if we dig around in the dirt of failure, we find the seeds of success. Our messy personhood, if we examine it closely, is about the illusions in our mind that we take to be solid, real, and the absolute truth about How Things Are.

The path toward a more healthy, focused, beneficial use of mind is life itself. We can start by simply setting up checkpoints in everyday life—such as getting out of bed, eating, drinking water, walking the dog—that help us remember to check in with our state of mind. When we change our relationship with our daily life experience via stewardship of mind, then the whole of life becomes a liberating experience. Ask yourself this one question: Do I want to be at peace, or do I not want to be at peace? The answer, in order to be effective, has to be unconditional. The response *"Of course I want to be at peace, but my partner is unfaithful and lies about it,"* is conditional. The translation of this statement is *"I want to be at peace, but not if my partner is unfaithful and lies about it. Then, I want to be miserable."* We have a deep-seated set of personal preferences that get in the way of a peaceful, focused, creative, productive mind. I'm not in any way suggesting that we stuff our feelings and deny that something painful occurred; we're simply *denying its power to affect or define us*. We less often resist what is.

Tending the mind creates a still center within the chaos of our wild world, like the eye of the hurricane. We're training in the art of peace and joy. We recognize that there's no promise that, due to our noble intentions, things will turn out swell all the time. This process of mind stewardship—of tending our mind—requires enormous patience. We have to do our best and at the same time give up all hope of fruition. Or as Don Juan shared with Carlos Castaneda, "Do everything as if it were the only thing in the world that matters, while all the time knowing that it doesn't matter at all."

We move toward difficulties rather than backing away. All that occurs— the good, the bad, and the ugly—is not only usable and workable, but becomes the journey itself. We can use all aspects of our life experience as a means for practicing mind stewardship—developing our mind into a bridge to the joyful heart that lives within us. What we do with our life is our unique gift to the world. The Ten Healing Practices, stress resilience, healing trauma, and emotional savvy are all powerful contributors to help us express our unique gifts. They help us develop clarity and focus in our mind, find emotional equanimity and compassion, and help us turn up our dimmer switch.

CHAPTER 8:

LIVE YOUR SPIRIT

"These bodies come to an end; but that vast embodied
Self is ageless, fathomless, eternal."

–THE *BHAGAVAD GITA*

In considering each of the three aspects of personhood—body, mind, and spirit—it becomes increasingly difficult to define each one separately. The body is fairly easy to conceptually wrap our head around; the mind is not quite so easy to define; and the spirit defies intellectualization. There are some concepts that we can *experience* but not *name* in a way that communicates their fullness. Such is the case with spirit; which means in this chapter, we seek to name the un-nameable. A challenging endeavor, indeed.

Before we attempt to name the un-nameable, let me say that this chapter is not going to be about God, in case that's what you think of when you think about spirit. For one thing, I wouldn't presume to be telling anyone anything about God. It's not my place to tell others about their particular belief. Further, I think the word *God* can be limiting because not all folks who believe in a higher power resonate with the word *God*. In truth, there's no word or grouping of words that can define or explain the indescribable organizing Energy of the universe. Words such as *God, Allah, Almighty, Jehovah, Father, Brahma, Christ* can mean a great deal to one person and nothing to another; no word can be an accurate reference point for what we're talking about here—language simply isn't vast enough.

So the real question is what word can we use here together to help us consider and experience That to which the word points? For our purposes here, I'll use **OETU**, an acronym for the Organizing Energy of the Universe. I'm intentionally using an unaffiliated acronym for our discussion in order to promote a starting point of inclusiveness among the 86–93 percent of our world that believes in a higher power. If you choose, you can also simply substitute in the word you're comfortable with when you see the acronym OETU.

Using the acronym OETU also assists us in moving away from the dogma that's been created around the various ideas of a higher power—all the judging and rules and the "he's good and she's evil" and "this one over here is a pure soul" and "that one over there is an impure soul" and "your historical records are wrong" and "mine are right" and all the seemingly endless iterations of polarizing dogma and resulting judgment that are squarely in the domain of human thinking. This dogma can mentally pull us further away from OETU, and from our spirit aspect, rather than closer. If instead, for the purpose of shared inquiry, we honor what the majority of the world believers believe, then we're talking about a higher power that organizes and instructs all that *is*. We're talking about the fact that a large majority of us are interested in honoring our personal relationship to something much larger than ourselves. So the real question is, what brings you in closer alignment with this OETU, in the way that you define it?

A good place to start is with spirit; and, sometimes the easiest way to start naming the un-nameable is to point out what it's not. Spirit is not a physical thing; we can't scratch it, cuddle it, or amputate it. Spirit is not our thinking or emotions; we can't feel happy, hateful, or depressed because of our spirit. Spirit is not related to our roles or jobs: parent, child, investment banker, sex worker, wife, plumber, sibling, friend, entrepreneur, homeowner, husband, philosopher, priest, celebrity, philanthropist, war lord, drug dealer, rabbi, life partner, politician, minister, dictator, environmentalist, husband, prisoner, or spiritual seeker. Spirit has nothing to do with the clubs and groups to which we belong, our possessions, our socioeconomic status, our education, our IQ, our EQ, our appearance, our talents, our belief systems, our family history, our personal history, our relationships, our hobbies and pastimes, our political affiliations, our country, or our religion. The Truth is, none of these things are YOU.

What *Is* Spirit?

Spirit is the vibration of OETU that becomes associated with a human. This means it can't be created or terminated, only transformed. It can't be good or bad. This Energy is eternal and always present. Indeed, spirit is the very essence of who we Are. It's the part of us that existed before we were born and that exists after our physical body shuts down in what we call death. It extends far beyond the realm of the little things we do in the little days of our little lives on our tiny spinning planet in our minuscule galaxy in this teeny-tiny corner of the universe.

Instead, our spirit is a droplet of the timeless power, Love, wisdom, and intelligence that's inherent in OETU, similar to how a droplet of ocean water is part of the ocean and is imbued with all the qualities of ocean. Our spirit aspect connects us to all of Planet Earth and universal life in ways that we've barely begun to understand, because OETU is the intelligence that throbs in each atom and every vibration that exists, matter and nonmatter alike. As spirit, we're not, individually or collectively, a static or separate system. Instead, we are a small part of OETU that has become associated with a physical being—a body. This body allows us to physically engage with this gorgeously abundant planet by learning, exploring, creating, and manifesting on the physical plane. Although spirit is eternally present, it can't be understood mentally, even though we're trying hard to do that in these pages. In a similar fashion to word choice around OETU, if the word *spirit* is one that will become limiting or barrier-creating for you in this discussion, please substitute the word of your choice—such as *soul, inner being, higher self*—that points to the idea of spirit.

Whether we're sensing our spirit aspect or not, as we walk, work, make love and create art, ride bikes, drink beer, sleep, hike mountains, watch TV, eat dinner, play poker, the OETU continually flows through us. As the French philosopher priest Pierre Teilhard de Chardin wrote, "We are not human beings having a spiritual experience, we are spiritual beings having a human experience." Our spirit is part of a complex web of Energy that informs all that *is*. Our spirit expresses through us as the Love (with a capital L)—divine power, wisdom, and intelligence—that is OETU. Which means we *are* Love. *You* are Love.

This Love is the nervous system this entire planet runs on, as well as all that lies beyond it. If I could choose one, and only one, thing for you to take away from this book, it would be this: you are Love in physical form. For all of my adoration of Food Sass, the miraculous human body, the power of the mind, the 97 percent of DNA that we have yet to understand, and personal responsibility—the thing that's most important is that we understand that we're Love embodied, and we're powerful beyond our wildest imagination.

The kind of Love that I'm referring to here is not an emotion or a sentiment. We have hundreds of different uses for the word *love,* from the love a parent feels for their child, to the love a surfer feels for her board, to the love I feel for chocolate. The **Love** we're talking about here is not that, but is instead the endless and pervading vibration of OETU that reveals itself to us in endless ways. It expresses itself in kindness, generosity, compassion, peace, intimacy, connection, we-first intelligence, joy, and empathy. We see it in the opening of a flower, the birth of a child, and in the relationship between the worm and the soil. Whether or not we recognize, honor, or cultivate it—we're connected to ourselves, connected to others, and connected to the deep pulse of Life in a way that can't be broken. We're here, in form on this planet, to live Love, connect, and co-create.

If you doubt this, I invite you to watch a baby, six months old and supported by a loving caregiver. Babies lead with the heart and show crazy delight about pretty much everything. If you smile at them, they positively beam back at you, looking you right in the eyes while waving their little arms and pumping their chubby legs. They're completely stoked about the whole connected interchange. They laugh with delight about the simplest things. They're as yet unaffected by self-doubt, cultural norms, socialization, expectations, perceived failure, and all the afflictions that can move us to close our hearts, close our minds, and cultivate fear. Fear, in many ways, is the opposite of Love.

In the core of our being, we are all living embodiments of Love. That's what spirit is. The fear that we learn and all the messy personhood that ensues hide the Love that we are. Our journey in overcoming our resistance to ourselves, in its essence, is to choose Love over fear more often. I'm not in any way suggesting that this is an easy task. However, choosing to align with the Love that's our birthright is the remedy to not only our personal life problems, but also to the relational problems of our species—families, businesses, politics, church, health, schools, and all of the various collective world stages on which we play out what's bubbling inside of us individually. It's the remedy that will support the continued existence of our species and our planet. It's the key to improving and expanding the quality of our experience while we're here, personally and collectively. Rabindranath Tagore, glorious Bengali polymath, Nobel laureate, and master of verse, wrote that "Love is the only reality and it is not a mere sentiment. It is the ultimate truth that lies at the heart of creation." Indeed it is. All that we want—Love, peace, joy, abundance—is already who we *are* in the spirit aspect of ourselves. Our life is an opportunity to express more of what's already inside us.

"Okay; that sounds good—more Love and spirit expression sounds like a good plan. So how do I work on my spirit?"

You don't. We can intentionally improve the health and balance of our body, and we can intentionally improve the use and clarity of our mind. Spirit, on the other hand, just *is*, in all its fullness and perfection, as a part of

OETU. We're all the same powerful and beautiful Energy at our core. With spirit, unlocking our potential lays in our increased alignment with, and expression of, this core aspect of our experience—as a result, not an activity.

The Dimmer Switch

All of us are spiritual beings of Love having a human experience in this beautiful, complex physical manifestation of life. Spirit is the light of OETU shining through us. Now, in order to play, create, and navigate upon this physical plane, the human package comes equipped with free will, an emotional GPS, and a **dimmer switch**, in addition to a body and mind. This "dimmer switch" controls the expression of our spirit. Just as some light fixtures can give off light anywhere from very brightly to very dim, based on the setting of their dimmer switch, so too, can our light— our spirit—be expressed very brightly to very dim.

Even though we all have the same OETU flowing through us as spirit, we're unique beings having a life experience that's different from any other person's who is, has been, or will be. Our free will and our use of mind, in concert with other important effectors like environment, create endless variations in our individual dimmer-switch settings—from person to person, and from moment to moment for the same person.

A person who is acting out as a serial killer has a light that's been turned way down on the dimmer; the light of their spirit is not shining through. The Energy of spirit, of Love, is still available, but the dimmer switch blocks it so it doesn't get expressed. A well-known historical example of this lowered dimmer-switch setting was Joseph Stalin, the ruthless Russian dictator. In contrast, a person who consistently speaks and acts with Love and compassion has a dimmer switch that's turned way up. Their dimmer switch is positioned so that the light of their spirit is readily expressed, like Mother Teresa, the Nobel Peace Prize-winning saint. We're all somewhere on the dimmer-switch continuum, expressing varying amounts of our spirit—of the Love that is OETU that we all have access to.

Our life situation is not necessarily indicative of our dimmer-switch setting. There are people who have awakened to their spirit aspect, turning up their dimmer switch, while sitting out a life sentence in prison for a heinous crime. Meanwhile, there are people with a lower dimmer-switch setting who are public figures with power over many—in business, politics, religion/spirituality—despite the continued far-reaching effects of their disconnection from who they *are*. When our dimmer switch is turned down by fear (the desire for power over others is simply another manifestation of fear), we're the perfect vehicle for heartless destruction. As our dimmer switch is turned up and we increasingly express our spirit aspect, we become a perfect vehicle for heart-centered creation. Expressing our spiritual self is not a competition or a goal; turning up our dimmer switch is a gradual opening, an awakening, an expansion of consciousness. By default, when we become more of who we *are*, we not only serve our evolution, we serve the evolution of consciousness as a whole.

"This sounds fabulous. Why don't we all turn our dimmer switches on high, right now?"

Because it can feel challenging. Turning up our dimmer switch means we must feel the world as the world truly is and accept ourselves in all our flawed majesty. Our full light has trouble shining through the armor that we build in an effort to not feel the world around us and to not reveal our messiness to others. We develop armor in many ways—with intelligence, anger, disengagement, fear, our power over others, or "being nice." Some of us build our armor as a big, swaggery show, with lots of talking, posturing, and drama about how important or busy we are. Some of us instead withdraw from the world. For the most part, we build the armor unconsciously, not realizing that, in addition to the pain and suffering we already feel, we're adding to it by isolating ourselves inside our armor. The dimmer switch can't be turned up if there's armor and continual movement, stimulation, and distraction. Our dimmer switch remains still if we don't regularly set aside a little time to contemplate, and to connect with ourselves and the world beyond the frenzy.

When we accept prevalent cultural ideas of psychological fear, competition, and scarcity, we're pulled away from the natural Love, collaboration, and abundance that turn up the healing power of our light, as we choose to move our dimmer switch. When we're constantly buying into the idea that we're not enough—whether because of our physical appearance, possessions, accomplishments, or our worth as a person isn't enough—we're completely missing the beauty, power, and perfection that's in each one of us, waiting to be turned up. The ideas of insular success and power are in direct opposition to our interconnectedness—the One-ness of all the manifestations of OETU—and stand in the way of us turning up our dimmer switch and embodying our true selves. In fact, not much in our everyday Western life feeds the spirit or encourages our journey into dimmer-switch-ology. Our culture, in this age of materialism, runs on fear and craving. Fear and craving are used to motivate people politically, socially, and economically. This means that turning up our dimmer switch—more fully expressing the vibrant, timeless, and empowered aspect of ourselves that has the power to heal ourselves and the world around us—must be an intentional act of trust and bravery.

Turning Up the Dimmer Switch

So how does one turn up their dimmer switch? The Ten Healing Practices were designed for the dimmer-switch odyssey. These practices—mindfulness, gratitude, humor, simplicity, generosity, perspective, meditation, humility, forgiveness, and remaining present—create calm and equanimity in the mind, which creates a more clear channel for the inflow of spirit. Mind as bridge. It's difficult to hear the song of our spirit through the noise of the world and through our distracted, stressed out, emotionally charged mind;

these act as barriers to us hearing and expressing that song. The Ten Healing Practices bring balance and integration to our mind, creating a receptive bridge that allows our spirit to shine through us more brightly, to facilitate our ability to raise our dimmer switch.

Raising our dimmer-switch setting requires that we loosen our resistance to the most powerful part of ourselves—our spirit aspect—and embrace our unfolding. We no longer resist life or the truth of our experience. When we look and see, really see, our armor, we also see that normally we attempt to solve our inner disturbances by protecting ourselves. Real transformation begins when we embrace our inner disturbances—our problems—as agents for growth. This is not an overnight kind of transformation. It's more of a leaning—from a closed heart to an open one; from fear to Love; from blame to personal responsibility; from shame to self-worth; from self-neglect to self-care; from isolation to vulnerability; from judgment to compassion; from me-focus to we-focus. A moment-to-moment leaning, where a greater expression of spirit is never perfect yet always possible. We lean into becoming more relaxed, joyful, curious, compassionate, connected, and open. To no longer resisting the majesty of our Truth.

The personal evolution that comes about from embracing an intentional, conscious dimmer-switch journey doesn't come about because you change your life. This evolution comes about because you change *how* you live the exact life experience that you're already living. How you do anything is how you do everything. Think of your daily life experience—working, filling your gas tank, nurturing romantic partnerships, procuring food, living with your family, navigating parenting challenges, coordinating social interactions and relationships—not as separate from your dimmer-switch odyssey but as the substance of it. We don't have to go hunting for opportunities to engage with the Ten Healing Practices and turn up our dimmer switch, they occur all by themselves, with astounding regularity, often in the form of "bad news."

As much as we don't want bad news or difficult situations, they can be important engines for positive change. These circumstances and people in our lives can act as triggers, can instead be good news, because our messy personhood daily experience is the perfect classroom for dimmer-switch-ology. If this seems like a tall order; it is. However, the dimmer-switch journey is one of a simple intention: to Love. The Ten Healing Practices are, in their essence, practices for intentionally living Love.

And how might living Love look, in the context of real life? It's certainly not always pretty or easy, so we must focus on being directionally correct. Meaning, over time, we slowly raise our dimmer-switch setting, living increasingly from a place of Love, knowing that any kind of progress, including our intentional evolution, often looks like two steps forward and one step back. This morning, someone might challenge your patience and you get angry with them in a nonproductive way. You might then respond by creating space, honoring your emotions, owning your mistakes, and generating generosity of heart. Later today, a similar situation won't trigger you, because in some small or large way, your earlier mindful and honest reflection primed your light for the future.

Some days, hours, minutes, I feel loving and gracious. Some days, I'm sulky and unforgiving all day. That's okay. There's an ancient teaching in the Buddhist philosophy that describes the dimmer-switch adventure as one where "before enlightenment, we **chop wood and carry water**; after enlightenment, we chop wood and carry water." I take this to mean that there's no before or after, nothing to achieve, and no big reveal; simply bring all that we think, say, and do to our expansion of consciousness—to turning up our dimmer switch—as often as we can remember to do so. This path is more horizontal (unconscious and slowly unfolding in nature) until it becomes more vertical (conscious and more rapidly unfolding) via all that we're exploring together.

Sure, some people experience radical shifts of consciousness—a massive increase in their dimmer switch seemingly overnight—often because they're on the brink of physical or emotional disaster. Their life is crashing down around them, or they're feeling depressed, or their addictions have brought them to their knees, and they have an awakening. Their recoveries are inspiring and make for wonderful stories and insights about the nature of spirit. My personal dimmer-switch journey, thus far, has not been one of intense crisis and a quick turnaround. For a long time, my personal evolution and dimmer-switch-ology were largely unconscious, until small and large life events started upping the ante. For most of us, raising our dimmer switches is less about a single life-altering event and more about a quiet, insistent internal unfolding, in the same way that an acorn must, simply must, become an oak tree—gently, quietly, and over time. Not despite the challenges of weather and water and insect infestation and soil quality, but because of those things. Growth and comfort don't typically coexist.

How do we choose Love over fear in such a polarized, emotionally charged, resource-imbalanced, and tricky human climate? How can we begin to function more consciously as human and spirit? As I write these words in the United States in 2019, I'm keenly aware that the overarching atmosphere is not one of Love and expression of spirit. As we've discussed, it's sometimes not easy to choose Love, nor is choosing Love a case of flipping a switch. The current environment is part of the reason many of us have armor. Many of us have been living from a place of fear for so long that it's hard to be a fish that can do a 180-degree turnabout to swim against the current.

Yet, the greatest power that we possess is the power to change our mind. We can always make a choice to see things differently. We can choose to live in fear and contraction, or we can choose to live in Love and expansion. This doesn't mean that we ignore our negative feelings. We need to feel them and learn from them, with the intention of moving through them and coming back to the Love that always resides in the core, eternal part of us. We live Love when we allow our most vulnerable and authentic selves to be seen and heard.

Choosing Love over fear requires courage and humility. Choosing Love asks that we relinquish the need to receive instant gratification for our efforts. It requires that we not make things personal and me-first, but instead focus on the universal and we-first. It involves respect of differences, including in race, gender expression, skin color, sexual orientation, religious affiliation, and political leaning. All of this can feel challenging to our dimmer-switch journey, but we must mindfully move through the discomfort. Choosing Love is juicy and liberating and sings with quiet, unbreakable resonance from somewhere deep inside of us. It connects us—truly connects us—to others in a way that nourishes and expands our heart. Love is an experience of spirit, just as wisdom and compassion are.

The Power of Compassion

Compassion, similar to many (all?) of the topics we've been contemplating together, is a Very Big Subject. There are many books written on compassion; there are increasingly numerous scientific studies on compassion; and some of the most wise teachers of our time—Mother Teresa, the 14th Dalai Lama, Thích Nhất Hạnh, Desmond Tutu, Maya Angelou—spent much of their lives as ambassadors for compassion. **Compassion** is the empathic desire to alleviate suffering; I think of it as the highest expression of Love, of spirit. It's a strong, empowered state that we can cultivate, regardless of our trauma, pain, or life experience. Compassion connects the *feeling* of empathy to *acts* of kindness, generosity, and understanding and comes to us through our spirit aspect. Compassion flows from the interconnectedness of all sentient beings and is part of the solution for our psychological suffering and our overall well-being. In short, compassion is actively wanting relief from suffering for self and other. Compassion is healing in the widest sense and it rocks our world personally and globally.

Despite the power in this expression of spirit, some confusion about compassion rattles around our mainstream thinking and vernacular. Interestingly, some folks think of compassion as weakness or wishy-washy-ness. Compassion is anything but weak and wishy-washy; it's a feature of a deep, powerful Love-infused strength that can and does move mountains. Folks also sometimes confuse empathy with compassion. Empathy is feeling with someone, while compassion is an expression of spirit. I'll step out of my math-geek closet and share a simple equation that explains the relationship between empathy and compassion:

$$(Empathy + Love) \times Action = Compassion$$

If we add Love to empathy and fuel them with action, we get compassion. The final confusion around compassion is that it's a Very Serious Subject. Compassion is beautiful and joyful, coming right through us from OETU, and play is one of the best settings for compassion to be expressed. Compassion *can* be serious, and it can also be playful.

Compassion is the subject of a growing body of scientific research, although we're just beginning to understand its power. Feeling, expressing, or receiving compassion elicits the release of serotonin—which regulates sleep, supports positive mood and healthy social functioning, and also combats depression—from our brain and gut. Compassion also elicits the release of endorphins and the hormone oxytocin. The former gives us the "runner's high" while the latter is protective for our cardiovascular system. Science also shows that the most potent effector on gene health and integrity is Love and compassion.

Recall our discussion about stress. Stress wears down the protective endings on our DNA, called *telomeres*. In addition to stress management and stress resilience, compassion is the remedy for our poor little telomeres. Compassion works to up-regulate telemoraze, an enzyme that repairs telomeres, protecting us from the damage that accelerates physiological aging, cancer, and disease. You heard me right; compassion rebuilds our DNA protectors.

Each aspect of our BodyMindSpirit affects the others and spirit is no exception. There's compelling research suggesting that we are wired for compassion, starting as infants seeking connection and compassion from a secure attachment figure. We learn compassion from this attachment figure, and we can even learn it later in life if that early attachment figure was unavailable. All bio-neuro-speak aside, the expression of compassion is healing for the body and mind of both the giver and the receiver; it's experienced in the mind of both parties as a type of psychotherapy. Although science is "proving" the benefits and outcomes of compassion, this state of being is at the very core of our humanity. It is vital.

This may sound fabulous and like a no-brainer solution to what ails us personally and globally. Compassion *is* powerful, and the world will indeed be a better place when more of us are living from a place of greater compassion. And relating to ourselves and to others compassionately can be a challenge. One challenge is that being present for people in pain, without pulling back in fear or disgust or anger or embarrassment, can be uncomfortable. Bearing witness to another's messiness or pain, without wanting to fade it or change it or fix it, is hard. Compassion isn't some kind of ideal that we're trying to live up to, nor is it a self-improvement project that we take on at New Year's. It's cultivating a new state of nurturing that involves giving compassion to ourselves as much as expressing it to others.

Being compassionate with others begins with having compassion for all those buried and unwanted parts of ourselves—all those messy personhood parts that we don't want to look at. This requires courage. If we're to cultivate the ability to care deeply about people who are fearful, angry, insecure, grieving, jealous, mired in addiction, arrogant, proud, Scrooge-like, violent, selfish, mean, you name it—we must learn to care deeply for ourselves. Because all of that is inside of us too, and judgment (of self or other) is the main barrier to compassion. Judgment dims our light. The trouble is that when we hit an emotion that's uncomfortable, our first instinct is to judge ourselves or someone else. The judgment is then often followed by shame and blame. When we aim this shame and blame at ourselves, we often bury it.

As long as we run from these qualities in ourselves and pretend they're not there, with our shiny exterior and our self-inflating social-media posts, we can't be compassionate for these qualities in others. What we love about others is usually what we love about ourselves. What we have intolerance for in others is most often a reflection of what we despise in ourselves. Until we turn and accept ourselves as messy and imperfect, it's nearly impossible to truly act with compassion toward the messy imperfection of others. It would be a rare person who is always compassionate, but if our dimmer-switch journey is real, we'll become more compassionate.

Compassion starts in noticing and understanding our same-ness, interconnectedness, and interdependence. In each one of us, there's softness and heart. Touching that soft spot in our heart has to be the starting place. To express the compassion that is part of our spirit aspect, we must start cultivating our ability to open-heartedly hold space for suffering and pain. Interestingly, simply naming something, from a place of Love, often takes the negative charge out of it: *"I can see that you're in so much pain, and I can only imagine what you must be feeling."* You see, compassion requires that we approach, understand, and connect with suffering. This, again, requires courage. It's well worth it. As one of the Kings of Compassion, the 14th Dalai Lama, has said, "If you want others to be happy, practice compassion. If you want to be happy, practice compassion." Our acts of compassion, however big or tiny, move us toward turning up our dimmer switch and living Love.

Live Your Spirit

We co-create our life experience, and life on Planet Earth, along with the OETU of which we are a part. We're conduits of OETU, via spirit, and we're creators on the physical and relational planes. We're here in physical form, hungry to connect, create, and experience. We're hungry for learning and expansion. We're hungry to, as Nietzsche eloquently said, become who we are. That, my friends, is living spirit. Becoming who we *are,* the Energy of Love. Living with less focus on our daily dramas and fears and more focus on living Love. Living our authentic truth. Relating to ourselves and others with compassion. Living our spirit. The challenge to each of us is our part in co-creation: will we create with reverence or with neglect? The center of the evolutionary process, on all levels, is this choice—it's the engine of our evolution. All that the human experience is about is the path toward wholeness and living Love.

As we fiddle with our dimmer switch setting via the Ten Healing Practices, living Love, and the power of compassion, the way we move through our daily take-out-the-garbage life shifts. The more-brightly-shining light of our spirit helps those around us notice their own dimmer switches. By increasing our focus on *how* we do what we do, whatever it is that we're doing, we affect others. Most *anything* can be done from a place of Love or a place of fear. With our every word and action, we're either expanding the Love in the world, or expanding the fear. We're teaching Love or teaching fear.

If we consider the people who've affected and taught us the most, it wasn't the information they gave us that caused our transformation. It was how they embodied the wisdom they were passing on, and how we felt in their presence. Maya Angelou, a Love ambassador, once said, "I've learned that people will forget what you said, people will forget what you did, but people will never forget how you made them feel." It matters *how* we do what we do. We are all teachers of Love in how we carry ourselves and in the quality of our being. We're not here on this tiny spinning planet to get stuff, prove ourselves, and find people to make us feel good about ourselves. We're here to turn up our dimmer switch and to connect, learn, and co-create with our human family. We're here to contribute and evolve.

As we evolve our consciousness—by prayer, by meditation, by the way we live and think and communicate, by our gratitude and mindfulness, by cultivating humility and perspective and generosity, by courageously developing compassion, by the lessons we learn in living this life with heart-centered intention—the way we see the world changes. It changes and changes and changes. No one is ever "finished." It's not like a thermometer that pops up when the Thanksgiving turkey is done. We must let go of the ideas of being "done" and "perfect" (that idea alone is a lifelong practice for me). We'll often be going through more challenges, learning in layers. This kind of shift is more akin to the long, slow turn of a giant freighter than to the turn-on-a-dime of a Jet Ski. It's an inner and outer practice. One that's vitally important for your health and joy, for your personal evolution, for the survival of our species, and for the health of our planet.

I'm sharing these musings not because I've mastered all of this, or because I live some charmed life of constant Love, nonjudgment, and bliss. The last thing we ever want to do is buy into the notion that spiritually focused lives and relationships are always serene, unicorn-and-rainbow-ish, and blissful. The truth is, we can't get to our truth or our turned-up dimmer switch by sitting in a sunny meadow; smiling beatifically; and avoiding our trauma, grief, anger, and whatever else makes up our brand of messy personhood. Our trauma, our grief, our anger—all of that is *the way* to our truth. Sometimes this messy personhood stuff is slimy and prickly and pathetic, but it's better to lean into all of that—talk about it and feel it and walk through it—and use it as fuel for our dimmer switch than to spend our lives being silently poisoned by our shame and loneliness.

Many also have the idea that becoming more spiritual means having mind-bending spiritual experiences where fantastical things happen, as if light shoots out of our eyeballs and we levitate. In fact, seeking extraordinary spiritual experiences can become yet another way to avoid our pain, fear, and resistance—or to make ourselves seem special—as opposed to an ordinary person embracing what's already inside us. Like compassion, spirit is also not a Very Serious Subject. We can just as easily laugh and play while we live spirit, as we can become serious or holier-than-thou. The former sounds way more fun to me. By bringing all that we encounter to our dimmer-switch path, we mindfully create our life experience. We're conduits of OETU and constructors on this physical planet—we're the master of our dimmer switch and the creators of our life experience. The path is uncharted. It comes into existence moment by moment and simultaneously drops away behind us.

I'm certainly on a dimmer-switch journey that's in-progress too, traversing that uncharted path, but I'll say this: when I lean into the Ten Healing Practices and dimmer-switch-ology, everything gets better. When I lean away from them, everything gets worse. For me and for everyone I come into contact with. The journey of conscious personal evolution is not an easy road, but once we've messed about on the road a bit, kicking some stones and checking out the scenery, it's impossible to turn back. Once we've Seen—gotten a taste for an intentional expression of our spirit aspect, and the infinite Love, joy, and compassion that comes with it—we can't un-See.

Who we are in this life is always a more vital teaching, and a more powerful transformer of the world, than what we say, and more essential even than what we do. As the wise sage Lao Tzu wrote, "Mastering others is strength. Mastering yourself is true power." That's what our discussion thus far—about habits and pillars, honoring the body, and tending the mind—has been all about. Increased alignment with, and expression of, spirit is the fruit, the culmination, of all that we've explored together. This mastering of ourselves—of becoming who we Are—brings us health and joy, yes. It's also the key to stitching up our wounded, wild world. That's right, you are the one we've been waiting for.

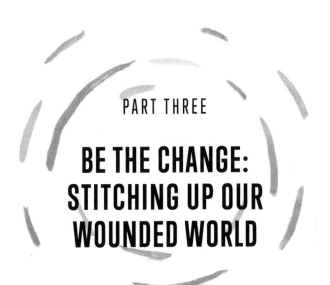

PART THREE

BE THE CHANGE: STITCHING UP OUR WOUNDED WORLD

We've covered a lot of ground during our exploration of how we might move toward the fullest, most vibrant version of ourselves. Reading about evolving into more health and joy can make choices sound easy, or at least simple. The living of it is more complex and can also feel challenging. What follows will look at this adventure through a broader lens.

We'll suss out how everyday unknown people—people like you and me—can create not only their own health and joy but also the health and joy of the collective on Earth. We're going to be thinking about how we can take our strides from the preceding pages and apply them to the larger intentional journey of stitching up our wounded world. Of creating a world where dimmer switches are encouraged to rise so that our lights shine more brightly.

Mahatma Gandhi, brave and tireless ambassador of India's nonviolent civil rights movement, said, "In a gentle way, you can shake the world. . . . You must be the change you wish to see in the world." Indeed, our history is peppered with inspiring folks whose commitment to Love famously changed the world, largely by the way they inhabited it, and I've mentioned many of them throughout our discussion. Maya Angelou, Thích Nhất Hạnh, Mother Teresa, the 14th Dalai Lama, Mahatma Gandhi, Pema Chödrön, and Martin Luther King, Jr. quickly pop into mind. There are others in our society such as influencer Oprah Winfrey, activist Colin Kaepernick, and research professor Brené Brown. Each are challenging our perspectives in important ways, opening up our minds to a fuller understanding of what it means to be human and to Love in our wild world. What isn't written up in our historical records, or typically covered in our news culture, are the everyday unknown people who are quietly working to stitch up our wounded world. Who are these people? What do they do? Why does it matter? These are important questions, and in this final leg of our adventure, they are exactly what we'll get curious about.

CHAPTER 9:

JOYFUL HEART AS CATALYST

"The most beautiful and profound emotion we can experience is the
sensation of the mystical. It is the sower of all true science. . . .
The scientist's religious feeling takes the form of rapturous amazement
at the harmony of natural law, which reveals an intelligence of such
superiority that, in comparison with it, the highest intelligence of
human beings is an utterly insignificant reflection. This feeling is
the guiding principle of his (or her) work."

—ALBERT EINSTEIN, "SCIENCE AND GOD,"
THE FORUM 83 (JUNE, 1930): 373.

One Is Infinity

Einstein's words above are pure poetry and truth and neatly tee up our discussion. Einstein is well known as a brilliant theoretical physicist; a science
philosopher; and a literal genius, with an IQ of 160 (a perfect score on the
Mensa quizzes is 162). What many don't know is that he was awed by the
mystical, as was the Indian mathematical genius Srinivasa Ramanujan. The
significant contributions of these two people to our knowledge and understanding came partly from their connection to a higher power. Many scientists, physicists, and mathematicians have found that science and spirituality

are woven from the same thread. Scientists find that when they're truly curious and open to what might be, their dimmer switch is activated. Spiritual icons, like the 14th Dalai Lama, often find that spirituality helps develop their fascination with science. This is interesting, as we often speak about science and spirituality as being at odds. However, the true scientist and the true spiritual explorer find themselves considering the same truth: everything is deeply interconnected. There is harmony and superior intelligence in natural law. The Organizing Energy of the Universe (OETU) instructs all that is.

The one that is you is a part of Infinity, and each instructs the other. Each of us is a part of a greater whole. We are 7.6 billion people knocking around the planet in various states of dimmer-switch expression. Our choices, our actions, our thoughts, our words, and our Energetic frequency *all* affect the people around us (society), the planet we all share, and all of the nonhuman inhabitants and physical matter that share the world with us. We are a working part of many nested systems. Our society—culture, politics, farming practices, waste management, education principles—affects us individually and affects our planet. Our planet—terrain, water, weather, natural resources, pollution, atmosphere—and all its nonhuman life forms in turn affect each of us individually as well as our society. This is *holism,* and it instructs all that has manifested on our planet, as well as all that lies beyond our little corner of the universe. Holism points to the continual elaborate dance of interconnection by honoring interacting wholes, as opposed to a collection of disparate parts. Quantum physics backs this up, often revealing how, even though we can't always see the connections, everything is deeply interconnected.

Backing up for a minute, the last part of this book outlined our body, mind, and spirit aspects as part of our BodyMindSpirit whole. We traversed each aspect, learning that the body is a staggeringly complex organism. The body is a fusion of atoms within molecules, molecules within the complex workings of a cell, cells within tissue, tissues comprising organs (such as the brain), organs as part of systems, systems that interrelate and balance—the nesting of parts seems to never end. The mind is massively complex in its own right as it instructs the body, acts as bridge or barrier for spirit, and profoundly affects and interacts with all that we come into contact with and much that is unseen.

Can you sense in your life an interconnected we as well as a personal me? Each of us is a tiny part of an elaborate universal dance of interconnection. Yet we view ourselves as separate. We've created these illusory walls of separation—between neighbors, towns, states, provinces, countries, religions, political parties, and on and on—which are arbitrary distinctions. We lose sight of how deeply bound to each other we all are—people, animals, insects, ocean life, viruses, geology, bacteria, weather, and all that's part of OETU. Together, we are the gazillions of "cells" that make up the organism of Earth.

The deep interconnectedness of all that is—everything we can recognize with our five senses, and everything that exists at finer vibrations than we have yet to sense—creates a web where the micro instructs the macro, the macro instructs the micro, and the never-ending iterations of this interplay shape our life experience. This idea, which wisdom traditions have supported for millennia, is starting to be studied. Indeed, some research has pointed to consciousness as being a global phenomenon that occurs everywhere in the body, and beyond—meaning that we're all interconnected by a field of consciousness, of mind.

At the beginning of this book, I mentioned that I think the most important thing about a person is how we move through the world, how we relate to ourselves and to others, and how we synthesize and assimilate the lessons and wisdom that naturally arise in our everyday, scrubbing-the-toilet lives. Our choices and our Energetic vibration—our Love and our fear, our kindness and our cruelty, our honesty and our treason, our mindful heart and our heartless mind, our self-worth and our self-disgust—touch everyone. This is awe-inspiring.

Indeed, when Einstein speaks about "rapturous amazement at the harmony of natural law," he is speaking about a deep humility-inspiring awe for all that is. He is referring to **reverence,** an attitude of honoring life in all its manifestations. When we approach all that is with reverence, we're honoring the value and sacredness of life on our planet, and beyond. I don't define reverence as synonymous with respect. Respect includes a judgment, and reverence is not about judgment. I don't respect mosquitos, because I live in New England and mosquitos not only can ruin a good outdoor gathering or a good night's sleep, but they can also carry disease. However, I do have reverence for the natural world, and that, by definition, includes mosquitos. Who am I to decide what's worthy or not in nature?

In reverence, we understand that there's consciousness in all of life—rocks, trees, elephants, humans, gazelles, apples, chickadees—and even mosquitos. A person in reverence cannot consider themselves superior to any other form of life because they see and honor OETU in all forms of life. As so aptly spoken by the voice of Divine Presence in the famous and historic spiritual text, the *Bhagavad Gita*, "He who is rooted in oneness realizes that I am in every being; wherever he goes, he remains in me."

Lessons from a Mosquito

Rooted in oneness, how can we make a difference in this wild world, which seems to be getting wilder? The answer: with our joyful heart.

We can create and live a joyful heart in a wild world, and our joyful heart can also help that very world evolve its dimmer-switch setting. Our personal evolution affects the Energetic evolution of the world. Before you resist that idea, I invite you to dance in step with me here, give a wink to curiosity from your Three Amigos, and see what you think. To this juncture, this book has been about you—about your health, joy, and personal evolution. We've perused the Three Pillars of personal responsibility, self-worth, and self-care. We applied those pillars, along with habits and the Three Amigos, to honoring the body, tending the mind, and living the spirit. We spoke at length about the Ten Healing Practices, which are central practices to all that we've explored together. We investigated the idea of our dimmer switch and how we might turn it up. This is all quite fabulous for us, as individuals—allowing us to create a philosophy and approach to life where we more fully enjoy and inhabit our daily life experience. We become more healthy, integrated, and Whole; and our dimmer switch shifts so our light brightens.

In the same way that one cell in my body informs the integrity of my body as a whole, one human can inform the integrity of the species, the planet. If I go into a dark room and put a candle in it, it adds a little bit of light. Quite a bit, for such a small flame. If I go into that same dark room and add ninety-nine more candles, it's like an overhead light has been turned on, with its dimmer-switch setting on high. Our joyful heart, our BodyMind-Spirit health, our integration and wholeness, and our dimmer-switch setting affect the world of which we are part, just like that candle flame in a dark room. In 1995, psychologist Daniel Goleman published his groundbreaking book *Emotional Intelligence*. When I read that book twenty-three years ago, I was struck by a story, and it sticks with me to this day. It was about a city bus driver whose irrepressible spirit and emotional intelligence affected the mood of everyone who had the good fortune to ride his bus each day. This was a Love bus (my words, not Daniel's). Pakistani education activist Malala Yousafzai is another example of how one person positively affects many; but you don't have to be world-famous to make a difference. One small being can create a big impact, simply by adjusting the dimmer switch that they carry with them through their days. Similar to a mosquito.

There's an African proverb that states, "If you think you're too small to make a difference, you haven't spent a night with a mosquito." As a girl who grew up in Maine, I have spent many, many nights with one singular mosquito. There are bumper stickers that Mainers have on their car reading: "Maine State Bird: The Mosquito." I can personally vouch that the African proverb is spot-on. Whether she was in my bedroom or in my tent, that tiny little insect could rob me of hours of sleep until I found her. She was either buzzing around my head or sinking her proboscis into my flesh—neither of which has a lullaby effect. Aside from the obvious suggestion of avoiding sleeping with a mosquito, my other suggestion is that you embrace your ability to make a difference in this wild world. Where to start? The fabulous news is that you're holding a whole book of suggestions. There's also a good place to start that we haven't yet specifically investigated: the power of honesty and kindness.

Honest and Kind: The Two Commandments

I know there are ten commandments in Christian doctrine; however, they're religion-specific and therefore won't resonate with everyone. The universal messages of the last six of the Judeo-Christian commandments can all be boiled down to: *"Be honest and be kind."* If we all practiced only these two things with *ourselves and with others*, our personal lives and our planet would move toward healing, joy, and connection. The trouble is, the Two Commandments are not *"Be honest and kind when it's easy,"* or *"Be honest and kind when it's convenient,"* or *"Be honest and kind to people who you like and agree with."* The Two Commandments ask us to be honest and kind as a consistent practice, including when it's uncomfortable. That's why these two simple words, in living them, aren't always easy.

Take honesty. There's evidence that the average person lies every ten minutes. Every ten minutes! This encompasses everything from huge whoppers to teeny tiny lies; and includes exaggeration, omission, white lies, and bullshitting. Most folks would likely describe me as an honest person, yet when I read this disturbing research years ago, I was intrigued and started paying close attention to honesty in my life. I learned that it can be hard to always tell the truth.

The first step in being truthful, as always, is awareness—noticing when we find ourselves deviating from the truth, or wanting to. Is that reliably effective in preventing lies? No. Are we consistently 100 percent honest?

Apparently not. But if we keep our intentions on being truthful—because we know it feels lousy to be lied to and that lying ultimately dishonors the fundamental integrity of connection—we can evolve the connection we have with people, and our connection within ourselves. Even the smallest of moves toward more integrity matter.

One snowy day, my then fifteen-year-old son, Alex, asked me to play chess with him. I enjoy chess but hadn't played in many years, so I was excited to play and to hang out with him. He set up the board while I did a quick review on my smartphone of how the various chess pieces are permitted to move. Still feeling rather rusty and clueless, I started the game by mimicking every pawn move he made. Alex, a competitive person by nature, expressed his annoyance at this tactic, as this sets the game up to reach a sort of stale-mate. Feeling a bit embarrassed, I decided to try a different move. I put my fingertips on a pawn and hung there for a second.

Alex: "You can't move that piece, Mom. It has no moves right now."

Me: "I know that."

Alex: "No you didn't. You were going to move it."

Me: "I was not!"

(Yes, I'm aware that I sound like I'm five years old in this part of the dialogue. Although this interchange with my son is a good example of how insidious lies are, and how they affect things, I can assure you that I'm not going to look amazingly mature and cool in this story.)

I started to systematically place my fingers on various pieces, hanging on each while considering my options.

Alex: "You're just doing that to cover up the fact that you were going to move that pawn, and that you don't know what you're doing."

Me: "No, I'm not! Don't sit there and tell me that you know what I'm thinking. You don't, and I know how pawns move."

Alex: [Stares at me with quiet disdain.]

The game went downhill from there and I felt ashamed and awful. Alex is a stickler for the truth and as I felt his resentment and my shame growing, I finally came clean about the whole darn thing, blurting out my confession: *"Alex, you're right. I totally lied to you a few minutes ago. I was embarrassed about my lack of chess savvy, and then annoyed with you getting up in my grill, and then I made it worse by lying. I'm sorry."*

This awkward story about a tiny white lie I told my son during a board game to save face on my chess ignorance illustrates two things: how insidious lying can be and how important honesty is. My honesty means the world to my son, and therefore to our relationship. I would say this is true for most relationships. Speaking the truth can be much harder than in the little story I just told. If we find that someone we care about, or someone in a position of power, has lied to us, it plants a seed in our mind that they're not always honest with us, and it's hard to know how far their dishonesty reaches. This feels pretty lousy. As is often the case, we start with awareness. Start by paying attention and by being willing to circle back and make things right, and please remember to be kind to yourself.

Let's consider the second commandment: kindness is an act, an intent, which has extraordinary power. **Kindness** is doing or communicating something, of our volition, that we hope will be of benefit to another(s) without expecting anything in return. Kindness has its roots in personal ethics and is a heartfelt concern for others and for ourselves. It's rooted in empathy and acceptance and comes from our integrity and our hearts; thus, it has a deeper meaning than simply smiling or opening the door for someone. Kindness isn't the same as "being nice." Being nice is more about how other people see us, about making ourselves look good; whereas kindness is based on our beliefs, ethics, and values. Kindness requires that we open our eyes, minds, hearts, and notice when others are suffering.

Kindness is a gorgeous, wonderful, and complex quality that has the potential to move our BodyMindSpirit life experience, and the life of this planet, to a more balanced, integral place. The great news is we don't have to agree—on anything—to be kind to one another. Again, when I say "kind," I'm not necessarily referring to acts of kindness such as donating to a charity or helping an elderly person across the road. These are certainly thoughtful and considerate acts. However, what I'm talking about here is something more integral: imbuing our daily words, thoughts, and actions with kindness. *Leading from the heart* in as many aspects of our mundane life as possible, whether or not we like or agree with someone else.

Kindness can feel easy and wonderful. Practicing kindness can also be challenging. Kindness often requires strength and courage.

Sometimes kindness means saying no, setting loving boundaries, or can even result in disappointing others. For instance, if someone is struggling with unhealthy behaviors, it's often kinder to let them face the consequences of their actions than to enable them to continue. With kindness, this decision to not act—to refuse to lend them money, bail them out of jail, or cover up for them at work—comes from a place of empathy and compassion, not of judgment or lack of caring. Being kind can sometimes be hard, especially when it means saying no, even from a place of heart. Having someone's best interest at heart doesn't always mean that we'll make them happy.

Similarly, it's less easy to express and live kindness when our feelings are hurt, when we're tired or hungry, when we don't like the other person much, or when the world is on our last nerve. Kindness, as a life philosophy, becomes challenging when waters get rough. Our close relationships can often be the most challenging for our desire and good intentions to act and speak with kindness. Anyone who has parented toddlers or teenagers knows that kindness gets hard in those trenches. Anyone who has been in a committed romantic partnership knows that sometimes unkind words, thoughts, and actions seem to take over. Providing care for, or being close to, an aging parent can also test our resolve to be kind.

For example, my mom is a healthy eighty-seven years old. She's a quiet, humble, independent, artistic, and loving person—I count my lucky stars every day that I get to be her daughter. In the last couple of years, since she had general anesthesia for surgery on a broken wrist, her memory and cognition have been compromised—a common but little-known condition called *postoperative cognitive dysfunction* or POCD. She's aware of it.

When a conversation or event transpires where this brain change is evident, it can trigger me. I can get impatient, and sometimes snap at her, saying, *"I already told you that,"* or some other unkind, unnecessary comment. It can be difficult to experience and witness our parents' aging process; we often project our fears onto them, or onto fellow caregivers, in a way that's hurtful. Psychological fear is a slippery bastard and can strain our intention to be kind.

The last time I snapped at my mom because she told me a story for the third time, I took a step back and was able to realize that I was acting out of fear—of her getting older, of change, of death—and I talked to her about it. As with everything, awareness is the place to start. With my mom, I apologized for my insensitivity and promised to think before I spoke like that again. With awareness, I could take the action of apologizing from the heart, and reaffirm my intention to be kind to her even when it feels hard.

Honesty and kindness are each important in their own right—and they're important as a package deal. Honesty without kindness can sometimes be downright mean: *"I didn't come to your party because I don't like you."* This is not the kind of honesty we're talking about. Similarly, kindness without honesty can manifest as flattery, sucking up, and BS-ing. Kindness and honesty can be hard, regardless of how simple it seems to read these words, understand them, and nod our heads. Regardless of what we want to believe about ourselves. Sai Baba of Shirdi, an Indian spiritual master, said, "Before you speak, ask yourself: Is it kind? Is it necessary? Is it true?

Does it improve on the silence?" I've thought of this saying many times and sometimes found that I didn't need to speak at all.

Please remember that kindness and honesty aren't yet another thing to judge ourselves and others by. Honesty and kindness are not something we attain and check off a list. They're intentions and practices that we commit to, knowing that there will be many, many times when we'll be dishonest and/or unkind. Please remember that you are not, nor will you ever be, perfect. True intention and practice is all we can ask of ourselves. Love yourself for trying.

The Two Commandments, honesty and kindness, combined with the Three Amigos of curiosity, awareness, and mindfulness, are powerful agents of change. The mere fact of our interconnection—which of course begets interdependence—can help us to realize why. In the same way that one tiny mosquito can make an impact in a big room, you can make an impact in the world. Within a life experience ruled by holism, your honesty and kindness are integral parts of a whole. Because we're interconnected, your joyful heart not only improves your life experience, it becomes a catalyst for a more compassionate and sane world. We can bring our health and joy, our honesty and kindness, and our expression of spirit to the greater planetary whole through mindful relating.

CHAPTER 10:

MINDFUL RELATING

"Our goal is to create a beloved community and this will require a qualitative
change in our souls as well as a quantitative change in our lives."
—MARTIN LUTHER KING, JR.

The personal journey that we've been considering in this book is inevitably
about Love and connection. All that we bring to our personal intention of
health, joy, and personal evolution comes home to roost in stitching up our
wounded world. We develop our personal responsibility, our self-worth, and
our self-care, deepening our connection to the fullness of our BodyMind-
Spirit experience. We connect to the majesty of our self-healing body, to the
vast and powerful tool of our mind, and to the Love that flows through us as
spirit. And we connect to one another—to the members of our human family. People are social animals, which means that our connection and interconnection are essential for us to survive and thrive.

Relationships offer us a powerful arena for healing, growth, and expansion. This opportunity also comes with a flip side. The opportunity for
growth through relationship exists *because* relating to people can carry a
powerful charge of Energy—that also makes it immensely challenging. We
often have trouble understanding one another and accepting differences. As
I write, America is experiencing a time of aggression and divisiveness, accompanied by communication wrought with pain, fear, and distrust. America is

not alone in this mess. Countries become divided for the same reason that brothers and sisters can become divided: people often seek power over one another. This desire to dominate others signals fear and self-loathing just below the surface. Relating more mindfully offers an opportunity for healing and authentic empowerment, as we look to more peacefully coexist and thrive on an increasingly crowded and richly textured planet.

Relating is about our connection with other people. How can we relate to others, regardless of the ups and downs that occur during our communication, in a way that fosters connection? We cultivate an inclusive approach focused on bridging, connecting, and considering all parties. We must bravely engage in dialogue with the intent to discover common ground, while honoring our differences. We need to decide that we're willing to do whatever it takes to keep the channel of communication open, and that we'll wait patiently if it closes. I call this mindful relating.

Mindful relating, at its heart, is the marriage of compassion and the Ten Healing Practices; it's woven into our everyday conversations and creates a fabric of connection, understanding, and shared experience. This is pivotally important for us all—lovers, parents, politicians, teachers, supervisors, workers, collaborators, healing facilitators, nurses—as we seek health and joy, personally and globally. Mindful relating focuses on the honoring of all parties involved—in a classroom, a family, a married couple, a company, or a country—and on strengthening connection, one of our most basic human needs.

We relate to others through all aspects of our BodyMindSpirit, with mind being the biggest contributor. Relating is, in its essence, an exploration—of ourselves, of one another, of our world, and of all of the topics that are important to us. Relating is co-creation.

I'll pull no punches here—relating can be hard. It brings us face to face with our core anxieties about ourselves, about our value as human beings. The great news is that if we can bring our vulnerability and presence to these core fears, we discover that the power of Love is much greater than the power of fear, and that any relationship can be transformed into a path of self-discovery by turning up our dimmer switch. We can start to truly understand how our fear-based attitudes blind us. We can become awakened on the micro level to who the person we're relating to really *is*; and on the macro level to how our mindless relating is playing out on a global scale in politics, religion, corporations, media, and more. If we set our intentions, we can improve and nurture what's arguably the most powerful aspect of personhood: connection.

Meaningful relationship lies right in that exquisite opaque space between "me" and "other." The zone where the flow of minds intermingle, where personal Energies mix to create something new—something based on *we* instead of *me*. This Energetic zone of communion is the powerful force that lies at the heart of human connection. This force, like most forces, can be a force of creation or a force of destruction. We move toward co-creation—toward synergy, collaboration, understanding, and Love—via relating mindfully. This involves an important shift from a *me-first* approach in communication to a *we-first* approach in communication.

Me-first relating is focused on ourselves—how can I most easily defend myself and get my way? **We-first relating** is shorthand for the paradigm shift that happens when we open up and get curious. Mindful relating is we-first communication: how can we best move toward a cohesive, integrated, balanced whole, even when hard decisions might need to be made? Using we-first relating can break the spell of focusing only on our personal agendas and awaken genuine relationships. It means that we can identify with the relationship itself, rather than with our individualism. When embracing the we-first approach, we can ask ourselves questions such as, "*If my words feel painful to my friend, or partner, or child, or those people-of-that-color, or people of that religion or nationality, how does this benefit me? Does it benefit anyone? Does it bring us closer together or further apart? Does it bring us closer to understanding?*"

If we accept that a one-to-one or group relationship can provide learning and the opportunity to evolve, these relationships become a mutual breeding ground to move us toward a more sane world. Starting right here in our home, office, schools, or on the subway. The key to enjoyable relationships, and to evolving our collective consciousness through relationships, is presence. We stay present with ourselves, with each other, and with the created bond of "we." By doing so, we may welcome the ups and downs of relationships instead of resisting them. We can approach relating—the good, the hard, and the ugly—as an opportunity to learn, heal, evolve, and thrive. In this chapter, we'll uncover the basics of nurturing connection through mindful relating. We'll start with what mindful relating *isn't*.

Disconnection Words

I have no idea who first quipped the words, *"Sticks and stones may break my bones, but words can never hurt me,"* but they were only half right. Words may not be able to break our bones or cause physical pain, but words are powerful indeed and we can feel deeply hurt by them. Words, and the communication that further powers those words—body language, tone, and intent—create impact. We've used words for thousands of years—written and spoken—to inspire, shame, celebrate, blame, marry, divorce, educate, rally, slander, parent, worship, entertain, and communicate love and devotion. Words can change the trajectory of a friendship, a business deal, a partnership, a marriage, an international alliance, or any other relationship where two or more people are in communication. Words can heal, and words can hurt.

In my childhood era (from 1966 to 1984), I think every kid was told the "sticks and stones" mantra , multiple times, by their parents and elders, when other kids were mean to them.

Me, in tears at age twelve: *"Mom, the boys are teasing me at school, calling me 'flatso.' They say it really loud in the halls and all the other kids laugh, and it's awful."*

The boys had taken the cruel insult "fatso" and added a letter to make it relevant to the fact that my hormones had not yet awoken, leaving me with the figure of a girl instead of a woman.

My mom, like millions of moms, would say something along the lines of, *"Oh, don't you worry about those boys. They like you; that's why they're teasing you. You're just a late bloomer! And remember: 'sticks and stones can break your bones, but words can never hurt you.'"*

I might've chosen a broken bone a month over that taunting. I'm not kidding, it felt awful—especially at an age when peer acceptance was pivotal. Painful words are often hard to forget, becoming deeply etched into our nonconscious mind as triggers. When we're the receiver of hurtful words, it can be hard to unhear them, even years or decades later. Let's say that Bill's father repeatedly called him "irresponsible" growing up, and then fifteen years later his wife calls him "irresponsible" during a discussion about finances. He'll be triggered. That word might have been festering untended in his nonconscious mind, and his wife's casual use of it in a discussion would act as a trigger, pulling all that old untended childhood pain up to the surface. Bill's reactions to his wife's choice of words might seem completely irrational and exaggerated in relation to the situation at hand, but his pain would be very real.

I'm not saying we blame our emotions on other people's words—that someone made us feel a certain way. Our emotions are our emotions. No one can make us feel anything. In the context of mindful relating—of intentionally creating communication bridges instead of barriers—we also honor that our choice of words can be impactful. Let's consider four words that carry a large potential impact, making them worthy of a spotlight focus in our discussion.

BUT

Our first word to consider is *but*. We explored the pitfalls of having a *big but* in the context of personal responsibility, and this word is worth a quick

review here. The definition of the conjunction *but* is that it is used to introduce something that contrasts with whatever phrase has preceded it, as in:
"I'm sorry I forgot to pick up your dry cleaning, but *that cleaner is out of my way
and my day was crazy-busy."* This is not actually an apology, in the true sense
of the word. Instead, it's something said from the Victim Mindset, blaming
an inconsiderate or irresponsible behavior on the location of the dry cleaner
and the busyness of the speaker's day. By definition, whatever comes after the
but negates whatever came before it. The conjunction can close our minds to
more inclusive thinking; and in these turbulent, divided times, we don't have
the luxury of short-changing opportunities for inclusive thinking.

Another way of communicating the same information about not getting
the dry cleaning, while maintaining the integrity of both sides of the sentence, is to replace *but* with the idea of *YesAnd: "(Yes) I'm sorry I forgot your
dry cleaning; (And) I'll plan my time better in the future."* It's amazing what
this small shift does to build connection and integrity. The apology keeps its
integrity, and the speaker is explaining and—the important part—*owning*
their behavior a bit too, which builds trust and respect.

SHOULD/SHOULDN'T

The word *should*, and its opposite, *shouldn't*, tend to bring out defensiveness in other people, while making us feel superior. The words *should* and
shouldn't often communicate subtle shame or blame about a person's choices,
words, behavior, or personhood. Here is an example in each of those four
areas, followed by alternative wording you could use:

Choices

Original: *"You* should *have taken the earlier bus; then we wouldn't be
running late for the show."*

Alternative: *"With your bus arriving at five pm, we may end up being late for the show."*

Words

Original: *"You* shouldn't *talk to your teacher that way."*

Alternative: *"When you talk to your teacher that way, it's received as disrespectful."*

Behavior

Original: *"You* shouldn't *gossip about people."*

Alternative: *"Gossiping is harmful to both the gossiper and the gossipee."*

Personhood

Original: *"You* should *show more initiative and work harder if you ever want to amount to anything."*

Alternative: *"Hard work and initiative help us reach our goals."*

Notice that the *should* statements feel like shame/blame and smack of an attack on someone's character, and the alternative wording simply states the facts, as they are perceived. This slight change in wording not only affects the person we're talking to but also changes our mental approach. We work to state the truth as we see it, as opposed to painting a person with shame or blame if they don't conform to our wishes or opinions. We keep in mind that what we think should happen often doesn't, and what we don't think should happen often does. Minimizing the use of *should* and *shouldn't* is especially powerful in improving relationships with kids, and within romantic partnerships.

ALWAYS/NEVER

Always and *never* typically communicate generalizations and labels. *"You never listen to me." "You always leave your clothes on the floor." "I never feel appreciated by you." "I always feel second-fiddle to your friends."*

Simply replacing the words *always* and *never* with words such as *sometimes, often, rarely,* or *occasionally* goes a long way toward helping the recipient feel that they're not being painted with a broad brushstroke of not-enough-ness. These alternatives help communicate that someone isn't always in the naughty zone, or never in the acceptable zone. And further, always/never statements are rarely true (notice that I used "rarely" instead of "never" there). My youngest son doesn't always leave his clothes on the floor, but he often does. I honor his efforts, regardless of how small, by instead using the word "often" in our conversation about him picking up after himself. *"You often leave your clothes on the floor and I'd like you to please pick up after yourself."*

NAME-CALLING

Our final disconnection word is actually a group of words that fall into one category: *name-calling.* Name-calling is pretty self-explanatory. It's when we say things such as, *"You're such a jerk,"* or *"Why do you have to be a dick?"* or *"Only a moron would think something like that,"* or *"You're such a manipulative bitch."* It's hard to imagine a situation when name-calling would inspire and strengthen connection. My guess is that name-calling has a zero percent hit rate in generating openness and vulnerability in communication. 'Nough said. Words are important, and so is the style in which we use them.

Disconnection Styles

As is so often the case on our journey, in order to fully appreciate why we might put in the effort for change—honoring our body, tending our mind, living our spirit, and practicing mindful relating—we first need to understand why the status quo isn't serving us. There are three *communication coping strategies* and four *me-first tactics* that hijack our ability to meaningfully connect. Each is a disconnected style of communication and has its own outcomes. Now, this discussion can feel uncomfortable for people. My hope is that, if you find yourself feeling the discomfort of *"Ugh. I do that,"* or an indignant *"Jeez, are we all supposed to frolic around smiling and being loving and tolerant all the time?"* that you muster up the awareness to notice your resistance or shame, and move into self-love and curiosity. There's no call for shame or defensiveness in the words that follow. Indeed, the words *strategies* and *tactics* can sound like a thing we intentionally do, like in business or in the armed forces, so please understand that these are not that kind of strategy or tactic. These are largely nonconscious habits that we use in me-first relating. We all struggle with these disconnection styles in varying combinations and degrees; many became part of our nonconscious programming in our childhood, like the strategies that we'll delve into first.

COMMUNICATION COPING STRATEGIES

Communication coping strategies sound helpful but are actually sources of disconnection. These strategies can include aggression (attacking), shutting down (withdrawing), and conforming to please. Conforming to please might seem innocuous, but it creates an illusion of complicity and agreement that both parties erroneously buy into. The former two most often have strong foundations in defensiveness; and, if we look closely, we see that the intent is not to communicate at all, but to punish the other and/or protect ourself. Although these closed communication strategies are born of nonconscious programming and perceived self-protection, they instead increase our feelings of distress and isolation as our connection to others is compromised.

Aggression

The **aggression coping strategy** is easy to spot due to its invasive nature, especially as we watch it play out on the world stage daily. Aggression is most destructive when we give ourselves permission to punish someone else for the pain we feel. Often, anger is fear or pain in disguise. The aggression coping strategy can include many "power-over" methods: shaming, blaming, name-calling, humiliation, and toxic certainty. Aggression depends heavily on self-deception. We believe that our aggressive tactics are sources of power in our relationships, when instead they're creating distance, fear, and isolation. Aggression can include physical aggression, as well as nonphysical aggression, such as shouting, threats, or verbal abuse. Anger can be an important and valuable messenger; however, it's our expression of anger that can cause disconnection, if we're leaning into physical aggression or aggressive words, tone, or body language.

Withdrawal

The **withdrawal coping strategy** is the flip side of aggression; often, mates that favor these opposing strategies are attracted to each other. For instance, my father favored aggression and my mother favored withdrawal. I ended up learning to withdraw for protection too and I still, to this day, have to struggle mightily to find my voice during disagreements with someone who favors an aggression coping strategy. I call it my armadillo response, and it's the favored coping strategy of my nonconscious mind. Although aggression looks more ugly from the outside, withdrawal can be just as psychologically damaging in relationships.

When a person withdraws, they are literally disconnecting. This can be confusing and frustrating to others, as they feel abandoned by the person withdrawing. The relational combination of aggression and withdrawing can be a wonderful opportunity for those involved to work together and find a middle way. However, if the mind is left untended, these opposing strategies can simply lead to exacerbation—the aggressor gets more aggressive and the withdrawer further shuts down.

Conforming to Please

The third coping strategy, **conforming to please**, is in some ways an iteration of the withdrawal coping strategy. Instead of meeting a person halfway, a person who conforms to please don't meet anyone at all. They simply say and do what will be pleasing to the other in order to avoid discussion or confrontation. If this person is a member of a school budget committee where the majority votes to cut back spending in the arts curriculum, they might choose to go along with the popular vote so as not to make waves. They hold back important thoughts that may have brought some needed balance back to the group mentality. Conforming to please is good for no one. Further, the trick is that, unlike withdrawing, when someone conforms to please, they appear to be in agreement, when most often they're in resentment. They might have opposing views and can't, or don't want to, express them—possibly because they've been taught that disagreement isn't nice or proper. Or maybe because it's how they navigated a parent or sibling who favored an aggression coping strategy.

These three strategies have their roots in a defensive stance. When we're defensive, barriers go up and block the flow of information from and to our environment, replacing it with our mental storylines, fears, and reactions. In the same way that Love and fear can't exist in a room together, neither can connection and defensiveness. When someone is defensive, they're focused on defending their wants and ideas. In addition to these three coping strategies, there are other, more subtle ways that we disconnect and shut down information flow, when relating: me-first tactics.

ME-FIRST TACTICS

In addition to coping strategies, there are several me-first tactics that we learn and adopt in our struggle to communicate with others. Four of the most common are *self-referencing, justification, projection,* and *toxic certainty.* Again, this is not intended to be an exhaustive discussion but instead to provide highlights of the ways in which we disconnect.

Self-Referencing

A common conversation tactic is **self-referencing**. Let's say I'm talking to my friend Ted and he's sharing the fact that he feels unappreciated by his boss at work. If he says one or two sentences and I immediately come back with, *"Oh, yes, I feel the same way. My boss, just last week . . .,"* all I'm doing is shifting the focus to me.

On some level I might be looking to show my understanding of his predicament; however, if I say more than a few sentences, then all I'm doing is shifting the focus to me. This typically results in the other person—who was dipping their toe into sharing and vulnerability—feeling shut down by my long diatribe about *my* experience. This can sabotage the flow of relating as the other person feels unheard. They may feel that we're not interested in being present for them in their experience of life.

Justification

Justification is when we employ mental tricks to support a self-deception that we had no choice but to do or say the yucky thing that we did or said. This tactic is closely related to the *big but* idea. Justification is similar to schlocky advertising that attempts to persuade us to eat junk food as if it were healthy, and to reject nourishing food because it takes more effort to prepare. If I told you that I lied to you because you often make me feel uncomfortable when I'm honest with you about feelings, that you left me no choice—that's justification. In truth, I did have a choice, it's just that one choice was easier and one was harder. Justification is the opposite of personal responsibility. There are seemingly endless ways that we justify our weak, unkind, inconsiderate, or otherwise-not-shiny moments by leaning on excuses, trying to justify our bad behavior.

Projection

A significant amount of negative energy in relationships can be liberated by dropping the tactic of **projection**. Projection means that we take our "stuff" (opinions, sense of low self-worth, parts of ourselves that we don't much like) and mentally or verbally wipe it all over other people, our environment, and the world. If I'm someone who experiences a lot of anger, I would experience the world as an angry place. If I'm someone who is a control freak, I would tend to have a difficult time around other controlling people: I would see myself and not like it.

We project what we don't like about ourselves onto the world around us, so that we can rail against it while still being defended. In relating between people, projection occurs when we attribute to others something that's true for ourselves. For example, a man might complain to me that he always ends up with passive girlfriends. If he were to own the projection, he might say, *"I've not learned to handle a relationship in which a woman is being powerful and equal, so I'm attracted to relationships with women who are passive."* A woman might complain that her partner dominates her and limits her. If she were to own the projection, she would say, *"I've not learned how to be my own boss and take up my full space in the world, so I attract men who want to dominate and control me."* Projection is a source of power struggles that eat up energy and intimacy. Projection is another way we trick ourselves into defending and protecting ourselves, instead of stepping into mindful relating with ourselves and others.

Toxic Certainty

Toxic certainty is the opposite of curiosity. It's a term used in Wayson Choy's work to denote expressing opinions as facts. It's being sure that we're right, with little ability to hear anything else. This is often accompanied by contempt for others, either privately or with our outside voice. Toxic certainty is having strong, unforgiving opinions about right and wrong that often come from a closed mind, a closed heart, or feelings of superiority—our belief that we have superior intellect, background, upbringing, religion, social status, emotional intelligence, and so on.

We have many ways in which we believe we're superior to others, and toxic certainty leaves no room for humility. Toxic certainty seeks to remove, or prove wrong, the input from others. *"Let's just focus on what's right: my view of the world."* Toxic certainty and the other disconnection tactics of self-referencing, justification, and projection keep our mind closed instead of open. In contrast, surrendering our defensive tactics makes genuine relating possible.

WHAT'S GOING ON HERE?

When we're using these various disconnection words, strategies, and tactics to wall ourselves off, we have only three preoccupations:

1. to get our needs met
2. to push away or punish anyone who threatens us
3. to ignore feedback

All of these approaches and preoccupations come from a me-first paradigm. They create and feed relationships rife with mindless relating. The truth is, if we pursue happiness, gratification, power, or control through relationships, we'll be disillusioned and disappointed again and again.

In addition to unraveling intimacy and connection, using me-first communication also serves to increase our internal distress. Instead of facing our fears directly—that we're misunderstood, unappreciated, unloved, unheard, or obsolete—we continue to push them down and focus on attacking, shutting out, or pleasing the other. The irony is that the very struggle to distance ourselves from our fear is exactly what keeps that fear in place, and then continues to feed it.

When we try to push away pain or fear, it most often ends up becoming a background anxiety, akin to an alarm that won't shut off. The physical and emotional energy taken up by this background anxiety keeps us locked in the secret fear that something is wrong with us. If we keep running and hiding, our demons keep chasing us.

Disconnection styles are nonconscious much of the time. This bears repeating. A first step in working with our disconnecting habits is to understand that most of them were programmed during our formative years; they're simply the relating tools that we're most familiar with. We don't usually enter into parenting, or a romantic relationship, or work on an important group project, saying, *"What can I say and do to protect myself and my own agenda? What can I do to annihilate the life-giving force of human connection?"* Sometimes this *is* intentional and conscious, but most often we're simply blundering through our interactions with others based on cues, habits, and behaviors that were stored in our nonconscious mind long ago.

It can be challenging to get our head up above this turbulent water and get a breath of fresh air. In the swirl of me-first relating, we can end up feeling lonely, the opposite of connected. Feeling lonely makes us emotionally hungry, so we look to other people to rescue or entertain us. We manipulate them to get what we need; but, because we can't possibly succeed, we invariably become disappointed with the people we thought might rescue us. We suffer, and we cause others to suffer. The opposite is also true. When we intentionally try to remain open and curious, to explore other perspectives, we can encourage openness and curiosity in others, which reinforces our efforts to remain open. Mindful relating can help.

Connection Foundations

Mindful relating is about communicating with others in a we-first way that fosters connection and integrity. It supports us, individually and globally, in navigating the challenges of human interaction when messy personhoods intermingle. Before we delve into the four cornerstones of mindful relating, let's peruse the foundational mindsets that lay the groundwork for success.

INTENTION

Intention is the starting point of every conversation and each interchange between us—whether it's 2 of us or 100 of us. **Intention** is how we direct our consciousness toward manifesting what we're aiming to create. Intention is the seed of our desire. When entering into a dialogue, it helps if, before we speak, we can ask ourselves, *"What is my intention in sharing this, or bringing this up? Am I looking for a particular response? What kind of outcome do I want?"* We can use these questions as a way of getting real with ourselves before committing energy to our all-powerful words.

When asking ourselves these questions, it's important to deeply inquire for the real answers. I recently asked myself these questions before a discussion with a close friend. When I asked myself the first question, *"What is my intention in bringing this up?"* my answer was *"To suss out where things went amuck."* When I asked myself the next question, *"Am I looking for a particular response?"* it turned out that sussing wasn't my pure intention, although that's the story I was telling myself. I was looking for a particular response—in this case, an apology.

If our intention going into a conversation is to make someone meet our expectations (such as apologizing), we're already moving into a closed conversation zone. An intention that encourages mindful relating, in this example with my friend, might be, *"I want to state how I felt her actions affected me, and to then be curious about what she was experiencing, so that we can work toward mending our rift."*

AN OPEN HEART

Mindful relating is difficult without an **open heart**. An open heart is not defended. It compassionately honors the messy personhood of others—along with ours—with a willingness to be curious and vulnerable. Roshi Joan Halifax, an American Zen Buddhist teacher, Zen priest, and anthropologist, said in her 2010 TEDWoman talk that, "It takes a strong back and a soft front to face the world."

A strong back means that our proverbial backbone is strong and supple; and, similar to a young tree rooted in the earth, we're grounded and empowered. With a strong back as our support, we can nurture a soft front. A soft front implies the willingness to be curious with our mind and vulnerable with our heart. Brené Brown is an expert in vulnerability, courage, shame, and empathy. She defines *vulnerability* in her book *Daring Greatly* as "uncertainty, risk, and emotional exposure—that is also the birthplace of love, belonging, joy, courage, empathy and creativity."

Through this practice of cultivating an open heart and vulnerability in relating, we find that our naked heart is more authentic and powerful than our masks and our armor. It also allows us to have necessary *boundaries* without constructing *barriers*.

BOUNDARIES

Boundaries are a function of love and respect, for ourselves and for others. They allow us to stand in who we are, while simultaneously honoring others. This doesn't necessarily mean *agreeing* with the other; we can disagree and still honor one another.

Barriers, however, are what we construct from a soft back and protected front, where we've turned the conversation into a me-first exchange. The barriers we build to protect us also shut down communication. Nothing can get through a barrier, in or out, as with the Great Wall of China. A *boundary* is more of a line in the sand, where curiosity and vulnerability are free to flow back and forth across the boundary. Keeping an open heart and allowing ourselves to be vulnerable can feel incredibly scary, but the Three Amigos can help.

THE THREE AMIGOS

The Three Amigos have accompanied us throughout our journey toward a joyful heart. And they most certainly are a part of the foundational mindsets that support mindful relating. The Amigos of awareness and mindfulness help us notice what's going on inside of us, and stay attuned with what seems to be going on for others. Awareness helps us move among the four cornerstones that follow, in support of we-first communication, as we notice the not-usually-noticed. It's important to remember throughout this adventure that the goal is *mindful* relating. Mindfulness helps us stay grounded in the current moment and is the undercurrent of all that follows in this chapter.

Finally, an open mind is important, which is another way of talking about our Amigo curiosity. Mindful relating invites us to meet whatever arises with curiosity. Instead of struggling against the force of confusion, we could meet it, relax, and be **curious**. I have found this idea extremely helpful when having disagreements with people, especially if I'm in disagreement with someone who's using an aggression coping strategy. When my autopilot starts the withdrawing into armadillo mode, I begin to feel confused and have trouble keeping track of what's coming at me and of what's going on inside of me. The force of confusion becomes large. So when I get the urge to curl up—which is definitely not mindful relating—I do my best to notice it and make an effort to simply meet the confusion with curiosity and relax. This isn't easy, but I'm increasingly successful. Simply thinking of the words *relax* and *curiosity* helps guide me.

Curiosity is especially helpful at keeping us out of toxic certainty. Eventually, as we work with curiosity, we find that we can no longer think of things as being completely right or completely wrong, because it turns out that things are a lot more slippery, playful, and gray-area-ish than that. Curiosity can begin with being willing and able to simply feel what we're going through as we listen to someone. If we aspire to stay curious about what we're feeling and what another is communicating, to recognize and acknowledge those things as best we can in each moment, we often find that something begins to change, deep inside us. We also find that under the surface of most conflicts, all parties of the conflict are people struggling with the same deeper questions, even if we can't access or verbalize it:

"Where in my life am I not telling the truth—to myself, to others?"

"Where in my life have I not kept my promises—-to myself, to others?"

"Where do I feel out of alignment?"

"Where do I feel attacked, misunderstood, and with inadequate boundaries?"

"What's keeping me from feeling complete and whole?"

"What emotions am I avoiding or not honoring?"

These we-first questions have their roots in curiosity and contribute to mindful relating, and to healing.

The curiosity of an open mind is the secret to a lot of things. It can take the idea of a "terrible mess" and turn it into more of an "interesting and challenging scenario." An open mind doesn't assume that we know where the other person is coming from, or even that we know what they're saying. An open mind is a place of humble curiosity. Part of the adventure of self-discovery in relation to mindful relating is lessons in humility. These lessons can occur when we notice how easily we slip into the very same things that we mentally put others down for. So when we feel disappointment, embarrassment, regret, hurt, insult, irritation, craving, and aversion—all the rough edges of our messy personhood—we invite curiosity. We can use them as stepping stones into reality instead of focusing on those feelings as a solid object that somehow defines either us or the other person. The Three Amigos, along with intention, open heart, and boundaries, set the stage for mindful relating.

Connected: Mindful Relating's Four Cornerstones

How do we relate in a way that fosters connection and understanding? How can we disagree in a way that isn't polarizing? What are the cornerstones to building and strengthening our connection? These are questions that have played on repeat in my mind over decades of navigating the difficulties of family life as a teenager, reading the news, building a marriage, working for companies, navigating a heart-centered divorce, parenting, stepparenting, working on teams, teaching, working with clients, communicating with teachers and peers in twenty years of formal education, and engaging with social groups.

My experience, research, and work with clients have uncovered four cornerstones of mindful relating. If this seems like a small number, in reality most people only think about two aspects of relating: speaking and listening. Further inquiry shows that the majority of us mostly think about speaking when we think about relating. We often think, *"What do I want to say to that person?"* as opposed to *"What might I learn about that person's experience?"* Speaking and listening are indeed two of the four mindful relating cornerstones. But, don't be misled by the limited space on the page that accommodates these two cornerstones. The fact is that all four of the mindful relating facets are equally important.

LISTENING

Being able to listen with attentive curiosity is the most important skill in mindful relating. It's also something that we are, in general, pretty abysmal at. Most people listen with the intent of responding, versus the intent of understanding. Say, for example, I'm having a cocktail with my friend Mary at a local restaurant. Mary is talking, sharing a difficult experience she had yesterday. I would likely start labeling, judging, comparing her experience to my experience, thinking about how something similar happened to me last week but also how it was way worse than what Mary is talking about. This would be my internal response to Mary's story while she's still talking. I'd also likely think about how much I dig Mary's shirt, wonder who's texting me as I hear the alerts on my phone, or try to identify a man who just came in whom I think I recognize from the gym.

You see, we're often either intent on our response or not paying attention at all, versus listening to what others are saying, and often we'll interrupt to share our response. Interrupting is definitely not listening, unless it's a carefully timed interruption to get clarification about what's being said, because we're being curious and want to understand something as fully as we can. Most of interrupting is simply interrupting. So what *is* listening?

The very best definition of listening I've ever heard is that *"Listening is the act of receiving what's being said, while opening to being changed by what you hear."* This is not how we typically listen. A part of listening is encouragement. Encouragement can simply be our attentiveness; it can also include a lean or head-tilt to the right, a signature of compassionate listening. It can be a gentle touch to a friend's hand or knee, or it can be a nod delivered with soft eyes. This communication of encouragement supports others in being vulnerable and true with their words, which deepens connection.

Listening doesn't take up much space on the page because it's simple in theory. The trick is that we need to understand what true listening is, and then we remain curious about, and focused on, what's being said. I'm not saying this is easy, but it's a main avenue to truly connecting with another via conversation. Also important is speaking.

SPEAKING

An important aspect of speaking, in the context of mindful relating, is what we don't say. Similar to my conversations with clients about food, where we start out with what to avoid, I spent a lot of our time together in the first half of this chapter sharing what's helpful to avoid when speaking—disconnection words and styles, communication coping strategies, and me-first tactics.

Beyond considering what to avoid, speaking in mindful relating is about two areas:

1. Be honest and be kind
2. Honor the Connection Foundations: intention, open heart, boundaries, and the Three Amigos

Years ago, I was attending a week-long training on speaking skills. My favorite part of that week was a half-day vulnerability workshop. I learned during that workshop that when we need to talk with someone about an aspect of our relationship that is difficult or upsetting for us, the words we use to communicate it significantly affect how our grievance is received. And, it's become clear to me, over time, that the words I use in my head also significantly affect how *I* see my grievance. It helps take me from Victim

Mentality to Creator Mentality, from toxic certainty to curiosity, from distracted listening to intentional listening, from barriers to bridges, and from a closed to an open heart.

Let's say I have a friend who spends a lot of time texting and checking social media when I'm with her. Let's also say that I don't like it.

Approach #1 (pre-workshop): *"Janyce, you're always on your freakin' phone when I'm with you. It really bugs me."*

Approach #2 (post-workshop): *"Janyce . . .*

I notice *that you're on your phone a lot when we're together.*

I imagine *that it's like scratching an itch for you and you simply aren't aware of how much you do it.*

Do I have that right?" (I practice mindful listening, preparing to be changed by what I hear.)

"I see. **I feel** *like I don't matter to you when you spend so much time on your phone when we're together—like you don't value our precious, infrequent time together. I end up feeling like I miss you when we're together, which is hard for me because we don't get to see each other that much."*

Pretty huge difference, eh? My gut reaction is sometimes to take approach #1, which most often lights the fires of defensiveness in the other person by focusing on their faults, screwups, or general wrongness-of-being. All of this squarely falls outside of the mindful relating zip code. Approach #2 achieves communication about the same issue, but nowhere in those words or intention am I attacking Janyce's choices or character. Instead, I focus on communicating my perspective of the experience while grounding my words and tone in kindness, curiosity, and vulnerability.

Is the second one more work? You bet it is. It's work to mindfully choose what's right and constructive over what's easy and potentially destructive. I have to think about what I'm trying to communicate and what my issue is. Because let's face it: it's my issue. A huge step toward a kinder, more compassionate use of words is to realize that when we have a problem, it's *our* problem. If it were a problem for the other person, they wouldn't be doing/saying the thing that we receive as a problem. Speaking and listening are conceptually simple. What typically makes them difficult are those powerful messengers, emotions.

EMOTIONS

Emotions are an important aspect of relating because they can help guide discussion toward authentic understanding and connection. Their potency can be helpful, and it can also be enormously destructive. The tripwire that creates our fall into destructive communication is *becoming* our emotions.

Emotions are an extensive topic. In the context of this discussion on mindful relating, we'll build on our prior discussion about emotional savvy. There are three concepts that can provide some touchpoints of support for using emotions as a useful, healthy aspect of relating: owning, honoring, and navigating emotions.

Own Your Emotions

Remember, your emotions are exactly that: your emotions. Our relating becomes more mindful when we remember not to blame our emotional reactions (messengers) or emotional swirling (our soil in our glass) on other people. Instead we own them as part of our navigation equipment and our learning. These approaches can reduce the intensity and discord that can make constructive relating so challenging.

Honor Your Emotions

Honoring emotions means that when emotions arise—for ourselves or for others—during a conversation or argument, we address the emotion, sit with it and let it soften, or we allow it to pass through. To be clear, this is the opposite of stuffing or ignoring emotion. Honoring emotions is when we turn our full attention to the emotion with curiosity and an open heart, allowing it to have its moment in the sun. What we often feel compelled to do is to dramatize, spread blame, and utilize the mindless relating tactic of self-justification. We unconsciously throw kerosene on our emotions so they will feel more real and so we can then emote and drag others into our emotion with us. On the other hand, we often attack, discount, or ridicule the emotions of others. All of this invariably goes not-so-well and breaks down the safe space we're working to create with mindful relating. Instead, we honor our emotions, and honor those of the other(s).

Navigate Your Emotions

Navigating emotions is about learning to ride the waves that can get roiled up in intense communication situations. We navigate the messengers and the soil with awareness, mindfulness, and intent. I've come to explain emotional navigation using the analogy of a traffic light.

Before you continue reading it might be helpful to review the section on emotional turbulence in Chapter 7. When I talk with people after they've read about emotional turbulence, they usually start to notice that people give cues about their emotional state. And they start to notice their own patterns and sensory cues in their body that communicate to us our state of receptivity and emotional integrity. Awareness of these cues helps us to navigate emotions in a way that supports connection instead of breaking connection down. Let's start by exploring how these cues might denote a red light.

RED LIGHT

It's important to learn to recognize the red-light signals for coping strategies and disconnection tactics, in ourselves and others, such as aggression, withdrawing, or justification. When we can see these signals, we know to stop instead of pushing forward into the danger zone. Stopping at a red light gives us the space to be curious and compassionate and to take a breathing snack. Just like in a car, plowing through the red light invites destruction in the form of destructive emotions—hatred, jealousy, aggression, anxiety, mania, jealousy, contempt—which are felt in the body as tension. These red-light emotions most often focus on past and future rather than the present; and, when ignored, they can become damaging. They tend to push us into me-first or win/lose and they make things worse the more we indulge them. Watch for shame, blame, name-calling, aggression, and justifying. These are all difficult emotions and tactics to navigate, for the speaker and for the listener, and are a red light in mindful relating.

YELLOW LIGHT

In mindful relating, a yellow light is the cautionary period of relating that's just before or just after the red light of communication shut-down. In these moments, maybe we've been caught off guard and feel a yellow-light emotion such as embarrassment, irritation, disappointment, doubt, frustration, fear, guilt, or feeling insulted. Below the surface of these reactions, deeper fears and self-doubts are becoming exposed through the dialogue. If we can meet these fears with gentle insight, using mindfulness practice, we can intercept our red-light triggers and cautiously move toward a green light. Small acts of kindness, either shared or withheld during yellow-light periods, can make or break a dialogue. Kindness, gentleness, and gratitude on both sides make our yellow-light reactions workable. The tricky part is that we tend to hide our yellow-light emotions, fearing that they'll prove that we're unlovable, unworthy, unforgivable, unwelcome, or powerless. Navigating the yellow light requires enormous presence and energy, along with plenty of patience and bravery.

GREEN LIGHT

Green light signals show that we can continue to move forward—that we're connected and moving in the direction of understanding, even if we're not in agreement. Here, we find ourselves experiencing states such as love, appreciation, empathy, joy, admiration, compassion, relief, and even alarm or sadness. These emotions lend themselves to bridging and typically come from a place of authentic emotion—from the reality of the combination of our inner landscape and what's externally transpiring.

It's important to remember that we can find the middle way between indulging and repressing red-light emotions by heeding yellow-light emotions, and by acknowledging whatever arises without judgment. Another important idea is that when emotions are in play, it's counterproductive to try to talk yourself or anyone else out of the emotions that arise. It's best to eliminate phrases like *"Please don't cry"* and *"What the hell are you crying about?"* and *"There's nothing to be angry about"* and *"That's certainly nothing to get upset about."* It would be a rare person who enjoys being told how to feel, so this type of dismissive statement is counterproductive. A better bet, if we're feeling oh-so-frustrated with another's emotional state, is to create space.

SPACE

Space in relating is vitally important; giving space, to others and to ourselves, is an essential part of navigating difficult conversations. We need pockets of space during mindful relating, and we often need space afterward as well—to reflect, process our emotions and thoughts, and decompress. This is especially the case when relating within the context of a close relationship. Our special relationships can stir up powerful transformative Energies, and we need plenty of space to integrate the rapid-fire stimulation that this kind of relationship can create.

My colleague Kim Barthel is co-author of *Conversations with a Rattlesnake*. Her expertise is extensive, including sensory processing and the neurobiology of attachment, abuse, and addiction. She taught me how to create space during a difficult conversation or group discussion while still honoring the other person(s). She explained that asking for space is simple and effective. Let's say that I've just heard something that leads to me feeling attacked or blamed, and I feel myself moving into armadillo mode. I'm at a tipping point between a constructive response and curling up in a ball—yellow light—and I need the conversation to slow down. I need space. I can say, *"This is really hard for me,"* or *"This is a lot to process and I'm really struggling right now."*

Saying these kind of things creates space for me, while still honoring the other(s). Knowing to ask for space is a crucial tool in navigating a yellow-light signal during mindful relating. Mindful relating does not require us to always be ready with some mindful, constructive response. Personhood is way more organic, messy, and challenging than that. Remember, this is about authentic, open-hearted communication as part of relation, not about perfection, quick responses, or some mindful relating grading system. Acknowledging that we need space is a healthy part of mindful relating, and sometimes our relational journey requires space in the form of silence.

Silence is underrated. In conversation, there's blank silence, and then there's attentive silence—a communing, processing, listening kind-of-silence. Attentive silence is more akin to communion with the ocean as we sit on a quiet beach, or communion with the earth as we walk the woods in solitude. In that absence of voice and noise, we can sometimes feel the OETU permeate our entire being. We can pause and release the need to fill the silence. In mindful relating, we can create space between the arising of an emotion—craving, loneliness, offense, aversion, despair—and the action/words that we contribute as a result. There's often something in that space that we don't want to experience—that we never do experience—because we act quickly to get past the uncomfortable feeling.

It can be a transformative experience to simply pause instead of immediately filling up the space. We become at home in the world when we become at home in ourselves. When we're here in the present, without anxiety about being perfect, we're liberated. In the silence during a challenging conversation, it's important to be clear to the other that we're not withdrawing: *"This is a lot to process and I'm struggling right now. Can we take a fifteen-minute break so I can get some fresh air and sort things out a bit?"*

Then, there's the space that can follow conversation when our conscious and nonconscious mind can sift things out a bit. I think of this as *reflective silence*. Sometimes that space finds us wanting to circle back to our mindful-relating partner(s) with new insights, questions, or discussion points. Especially when we make mistakes, our tendency is to deny them, to ourselves and others, and sweep them under the rug. Instead, in the context of mindful relating, we can go to someone and say, *"Hey, that thing I did/ said last week was bad behavior on my part. I tend to get triggered when ___ happens. I see it now and am going to do my best to do better, going forward."* This type of mistake-owning is healing to the other person and is healing to us. It builds deep trust in the relationship. When the going gets rough, we take some space and breathe, calling on our mindfulness practice to help us ground in the present moment.

Tending the Magic

Relating to others can be beautiful, enjoyable, and instructive—and it can also be challenging. Mindful relating can be intense for people, and there's no way around that. It's possible that you're feeling a tad overwhelmed. How to start? The easiest way to lean into mindful relating is to focus on incorporating the Two Commandments into your intention and dialogue: be honest and kind. You'll notice that the majority of me-first relating styles—disconnection words and styles, communication coping strategies, and me-first tactics—are naturally eliminated when our intention is to be honest and kind. Even if—especially if—we're in disagreement or feeling triggered. Being honest and kind is a splendid way to micromovement into mindful relating.

The tips and information I've shared in this chapter can help you understand what's going on below the surface during communication. To see that we naturally bring our messy personhood—our old wiring, our wounds, our shame, and our insecurities—to relating with others. Our messiness is par for the course and it also provides a solid individual training ground for mindful relating.

So far our discussion on relating has been focused on the relating that goes on between people. Mindful relating can also improve our pillar of self-worth when we apply these ideas to how we talk to *ourselves* in the privacy of our mind. You may have heard the saying that we can't truly love anyone else until we learn to love ourselves. In my experience, this is largely true. Similarly, relating to *ourselves* mindfully and compassionately is often a challenge. Learning to do so can open the door to seeing value in others and to relating with them more mindfully. Most often, the words we use with others are simply a reflection of the words we use in our mind. When we become more kind and accepting of ourselves in our inner dialogue, this will naturally spread to our words with others.

I experienced this concept in action when I was spending an hourlong coaching session with a young woman at one of the companies I consult for. She had struggled for most of her life with various kinds of eating disorders. It took about seven minutes to notice a theme in the way she talked to herself. Right after she said, " . . . and I totally suck at healthy snack choices," I pointed out what she just said. I also shared that I'd heard similar unkindnesses several times when she was talking.

Me: "Emily, you don't have your own back. You have to start there. Instead of 'I totally suck at healthy snack choices,' maybe try 'Eating healthy snacks is a challenge for me' or 'I struggle with making healthy snack choices' or 'Whew! Boy oh boy, is coming up with healthy snack choices HARD.' Do you hear the difference?"

At this point, she was staring at me with big eyes and I couldn't figure out if she thought I was off my rocker, or if what I was saying was making some sense to her. After a few moments of silence, she responded.

Emily: "Wow, I've never noticed. What else did I say like that?"

Me: "Good! Noticing and awareness are important first steps in any change. Your inner voice is actually more important than your food choices right now. We'll definitely talk about the food in a few minutes, but to answer your question, in the very beginning of our time together, you mentioned being stressed in your job because you're 'a complete failure at cold calling.'"

Emily: "Whoa. I did say that, didn't I? It sounds sad—sorta mean—when I hear it repeated back to me."

Me: "Yes, and that's genius that you're hearing it! Let's break that down into more usable parts. First off, most people are horrible at cold calling because, for the majority of people, it's a difficult and demoralizing task. When I was working in inside sales during my days in high tech, I loathed cold calling with every fiber of my being. So, step one in breaking that down is that it's not personal to you; it's actually pretty universal."

Emily: "It is?! This is my first job out of college and I thought my issues were because I'm not cut out for this job and that I would have to rethink my whole career plan."

Me: "Well, the first step is to give yourself a chance. Let's change up the words you use with yourself. Instead of 'I'm a failure at cold calling,' try this on for size:

'**I notice that** cold calling is a challenge for me.'

'**I imagine that** my boss also notices this and feels I should do better at it, in order to meet my quota each month. And she would be right.'

'**I feel that** I like most of my job and I want to excel, so I'm going to discuss this with my boss and ask if there's training I can do to improve my cold-calling skills and my comfort with it.'"

Do those bolded word choices sound familiar? They're straight out of the "speaking" cornerstone of our discussion on mindful relating; we speak to ourselves in our heads all the time. Emily had never noticed the way the voice in her head sounded, so this insight and her willingness to work with it supported her in making some important changes over time—in her job skills and her challenges with eating disorders. Now, when she emails me with questions or updates, she'll write things such as, *"I continue to be challenged by sugar cravings. Any thoughts?"* Choosing our words mindfully and using the tools of mindful relating—with others and with ourselves—paves the way for joy, personal evolution, and a more sane world.

Mindful relating is vitally important and has the power to change everything—from school classrooms to marriages to family relationships to boardroom conversations to the political arena to law enforcement—it can affect change anywhere we relate. This is fabulous news. It's also true that mindfully working to override old relational patterns and engaging from a place of vulnerability and curiosity is hard. We're asking ourselves to let the Energy of the emotion pierce us to the heart and open us, rather than harden ourselves by numbing our emotions or running from them. Plus, we have to navigate the shifting waters of dialogue and connection while we do all that. Mindful relating takes fortitude and courage.

Working with mindful relating is the path of compassion—the path of cultivating bravery and whole-heartedness. With kindness, honesty, and respect, we intentionally honor and support our differences—our *differentiation*—while upholding and developing our connection—our *integration*. Both differentiation and integration are the keys to balance, health, and wholeness at all levels of life. Mustering up the courage for mindful relating, as often as we're able, can engage us in true connection, one of the most powerful healing forces we know.

You likely noticed the Ten Healing Practices are woven throughout this mindful relating discussion, including mindfulness, the present, gratitude, perspective, and humility. The Ten Healing Practices are foundational to everything in this book because our mind is the tool that shapes our life experience. If, for instance, I practice forgiveness with others and myself, this supports mindful relating. These ten practices help our ability to relate mindfully, and relating mindfully helps us to develop these ten practices.

There's no need to wait for the perfect opportunity to practice. Mindful relating is a *chop wood and carry water* endeavor. It's in the subtleties of our daily mundane lives that we learn to relate mindfully. No need to wait for a Big Conversation. Start with the everyday small ones. Try it with the person who cut in front of you in the ticket line or with your son who just got detention in school or when your neighbor lets her dog crap in your yard for the 94,000th time. In practice, these keys, guideposts, and suggestions are less about analyzing ourselves and more about fully showing up in relationship.

I'll say it again: similar to many of the ideas and philosophies in this book, mindful relating is deceptively easy to talk about while exquisitely challenging to put into action. I'm saying it again because my hope is that you won't feel defeated when conversations don't go perfectly after you read this chapter. When strong emotions come up, all the doctrines and beliefs we've assembled for ourselves seem kind of pitiful in comparison to those large-and-in-charge emotions. Keep heart, love yourself for trying, and remember that perfection is the enemy of progress. Practicing mindful relating helps us stay healthy, even beyond the mindful-relating arena where we engage with others. Mindful relating allows us to strengthen our emotional savvy so that we're less affected by the small, daily life challenges and better poised to navigate the big challenges with more grace, connection, and courage. This emotional savvy turns down the volume on our drama and helps us tune in to whatever is going on in the present moment, whether it's comfortable or not.

As our life experience becomes more peaceful and joyful and our dimmer switch turns our light increasingly brighter, we're healing our personal experience—and the experience of humanity at large. Relating from a place of mindfulness, with the heart intent on connection, contains the power to change the world in a fundamental and positive way. With every brave conversation that we have, we evolve the way in which we move through the world, shifting our wild world toward sanity.

CHAPTER 11:

WILD WORLD GONE SANE

We evolve for ourselves, and we evolve
on behalf of life itself.
The full majesty of our empowered well-being
is the answer to all our prayers.

Creating health and joy in a wild world is a courageous journey. It's a journey about you and a journey about us all, and each of us has a unique path to walk. As you consider the personal evolution buffet that's been laid out in this book, I invite you to move toward what you feel most hungry for.

What are you hungry for? What is the one thing that you find yourself most excited about? Is it habits and rewiring the nonconscious mind? Maybe it's the Three Amigos or the Two Commandments. Maybe it's self-worth, self-care, or personal responsibility. Perhaps your physical well-being is top-of-mind for you and you are wanting a nutrient-dense breakfast to start your days with some Food Sass. Possibly you're intrigued with the idea that the mind is either a bridge or a barrier to everything in your experience. Maybe you'll start with developing stress-management habits. Or, perhaps you'll experiment with the idea that your emotions are the personal messengers of your innate GPS. For some, the Ten Healing Practices are what they've been waiting for as a gateway to a more vibrant, meaningful life experience. Others will feel uncomfortable resonance (welcome to the club) with some of the disconnection styles and work with the four cornerstones of mindful relating. Maybe you're still thinking about the power of Love and compassion and are interested in turning up your dimmer switch. There is so much opportunity for us to create the health and joy that we desire. What a feast!

Of course, all of these things are interrelated. In many ways, by leaning into one thing, you're leaning into them all. That's the beauty of being a sentient, complex, physical being who vibrates with the power of OETU each and every second. We keep one foot in our enough-ness and the other in intentional evolution, loving ourselves as we are, while engaging in the co-creation dance that's our birthright. You see, in addition to co-creating by manifesting physical things and intellectual expansion—wheels, E=mc², skyscrapers, smartphones, the study of biochemistry, paper, cars, solar panels, and rocket ships—we co-create ourselves and each other. It's part of the joy and pain of being alive. Before we part ways, I'll take the liberty of offering up some final thoughts that can guide your empowered journey to the healthy, joyful heart of being human.

Unicorn Trouble

Early in this book, we got clear on the meaning of joy. Joy is an important word, and it's a state of being that comes from deep within us and isn't predicated on external circumstances. Joy can come from finally understanding that balance is not a destination—it's a homeodynamic state, not a homeostatic one. In Latin, *homeo* means "similar to." Meanwhile, *stasis* means "standing still," whereas *dynamic* means "able to change and adapt." Our health and joy don't come from staying static; they come from our masterful ability to integrate and adapt. Think of a hawk soaring on air currents, and how he changes and adapts his wings and body by the second, in order to stay soaring. If he simply set his wings and thought, *"There, this works and I'll keep my wings here to stay in flight,"* he'd be in a heap on the ground within seconds.

He knows that he must constantly respond to external forces by adjusting his body positioning and mechanics. We're not hawks in flight, but are people with a vast array of external and internal forces that can tip us out of our homeodynamic state of balance—in body, in mind, and in our expression of spirit. Charles Darwin's theory was that the most adaptable survive. The balance and integration involved in creating health and joy requires continual change and adaptation. This also rules out the idea of perfection, which warrants a revisit here.

Perfection is a myth and chasing it will make you unhappy. We think that when we get to perfection, then we'll at last be happy and feel accepted—by ourselves and others. We'll finally feel worthwhile. This is akin to thinking that when we finally catch a unicorn in the woods, our life will magically be better. First off, most recent reports suggest that the unicorn, just like perfection, doesn't exist. This certainly makes for a long chase in the woods. But let's say that there is a unicorn, and you're chasing it. A person is not capable of catching a horse—horned or otherwise, especially with the whole magical factor added on—by pursuing it on foot. Even if you were able to keep up with it, you'd still have to stop and rest a lot because horses are really super fast. You'd probably spend a lot of time pretty discouraged and out of breath. No matter how you slice it, you'd be chasing a myth, and then feeling badly about yourself when you couldn't catch it. When laid out like that, it seems like a real drag, right? The pursuit of perfection is indeed a drag.

Releasing the idea of perfection doesn't mean that you can't have goals and aspirations to move toward. We all do. It's simply an adjustment of *how* we move toward them—our inner approach—and our expectations of ourselves while we do it. Instead of holding ourselves up against a rigid ideal, with self-flagellation at each misstep, we can soften our heart and look for opportunities to enjoy what we're doing in this moment. We live more in the present. Instead of crying over spilled milk and berating ourselves for spilling it, we notice that the milk spilled, smile at our clumsiness (this is an important step); even more, we're happy that we know how to clean it up and feel good that we made peace with what is. This same process can be applied when we have a fight with a partner, the car gets totaled, or we go bankrupt. The secret is your mindset. Again, I'm not saying it's easy, because we can become so darn accustomed to striving for perfection that any misstep, big or small, can lead to us feeling like that misstep *represents who we are*. It doesn't. Perfection doesn't exist, and we're so much more than our spilled milk. Failures, big and small, are simply events in our lives—they don't define us. It's all part of the journey.

What does matter, in any journey, is consistency. Consistency trumps the pursuit of perfection, every time. Instead of trying to eat perfectly or meditate each day with a completely laser-focused mind, we focus on being consistent. We might start by saying that we're going to eat one extra serving of vegetables each day, then create structure around the shopping and preparation of veggies to make our new habit easy. After we stick with that for a month or two, we'll have developed a habit. Now and again, we might slack off, because we're just perfectly imperfect that way. Maybe we'll have a particularly busy week, or there's a snowstorm so we can't go food shopping, or we go on vacation, or we get pneumonia and are on the couch for a week. Imbalance cropping up is a solidly dependable part of life. When we notice that we've slacked off, we simply reset and get back to our intention to eat a daily extra serving of veggies. This *is* consistency—a continual process that we amend and shift as life changes. Whatever you choose from the health and joy buffet offered in this book, consistency will be your friend.

No Right Choice

One thing that trips us up, as we build a life of intentional evolution, is the idea of a *right choice*. Much of the time, there's no right choice, simply different choices. Personhood is way messier, flexible, and forgiving than a One-Right-Choice option. Being a person is more about exploring options and taking steps in the direction that seems to be the best one for us. During the first thirty-four years of my life, I felt more angst about decisions than was necessary. Growing up, one of our family values was "no quitting." If I signed up for sport or a job or a class, I was required to see it through, even if I absolutely despised it. I do think that perseverance is a good basic value and am grateful to have learned it, but somewhere along the way it became rigid in my mind. I had connected my value as a person with my ability to make a choice and never quit.

This resulted, for me, in angst. I worried about making the right choice, had stress and sleepless nights, and sometimes ended up with analysis paralysis. *"I don't know which path to take, so I'm just going to sit down at this fork in the road and stress out about the fact that I'm sitting here."* This is an option, of course, but usually the reason we're considering options in the first place is that we want to move toward something, or away from something, or both, and sitting in one place implies no movement. I would sometimes put ridiculous weight on the simplest decisions. At thirty-four, when I had to make a decision about whether to go back to work or stay home with my newborn, I had a moment of insight—what I sometimes call a Moment.

A Moment is when we're going along viewing something one way, and then something sparks a realization that this was only our perspective, and that lots and lots of people do things entirely differently and, poof! We wake up to a wider perspective.

A Moment can happen during a conversation, while reading a book, watching a TV show or movie, meditating, people watching, and in many other ways. I love Moments, even though sometimes they can feel hard— it's often painful to realize that all along, our problem was our limited perspective (which it most often is).

When I was thirty-four, I gave birth to my first biological child, Connor, and I was smitten beyond words. At the time, I was a dozen years into building a career for myself in high tech and was working about seventy hours a week at a lucrative job. Up until the birth of my son, this had all been Very Important to me. Since I was lucky enough to have options, I was now facing the decision of whether to stay home with my son or go back to work. It was a nice problem to have, and I somehow still managed to turn it into a plague that haunted me for the three months of my maternity leave. As the eleventh hour was approaching, my mind oscillated between one choice or the other, multiple times a day.

At some point during these machinations, my then-husband, who also worked in high tech, looked at me and said, *"Laur, just decide what you want to try first. This isn't an irrevocable choice."* I remember staring at him in that Moment. My mind softened, and my heart softened, and I said something genius like, *"Oh."* I realized I could view choices as "something you tried."

This idea was revolutionary for me, in the way I relate to myself and others—and I still work with this concept today. I didn't, in that Moment, as we sat on the world's ugliest floral couch in a Boston suburb, say, *"Oh, okay, box checked; from now on I will view everything with less do-or-die edge."* Even then, I knew it was going to be a slow change, and I also knew that it was worth the mental and emotional investment it would take to encourage the evolution of my mind.

I went back to work. It ended up being a good choice because, after four months, I was able to see clearly that the best choice for me and for my family, at that time, was to shift focus back to home life. I changed my mind. I quit my job. And, because I consequently found 24/7 with young children to be challenging, I started leaning into my passion for Food Sass and health in a serious way. I began educating myself, volunteering with a nutrition nonprofit, lecturing around Greater Boston, and eventually earned my graduate degree. That time after I quit my job was when I started leaning heavily into my passion for human healing, health, and joy. Thank goodness I'd realized there's no right choice.

Over time, I've learned to challenge and soften my black-and-white thinking. Back then, I thought it was all or nothing: work seventy hours a week or none at all. Now, I cheer on my oldest stepdaughter, Jen, as she has remained in her career after the birth of both of my grandchildren, working thirty-five hours a week. It's a good balance for her and her family.

In retrospect, I wouldn't change a thing about my choices, because I like the present; and all that comprises my past has led me right here. There are many more nuanced shades and colors in our world than we typically see at first glance, and there are many rich and interesting paths to be curious about. The art of personhood is so much more deliciously fluid and forgiving than we allow ourselves to believe. I hope that as you eye the Health and Joy Buffet, you'll be curious and gentle with yourself, knowing that there is no right choice.

Learning in Layers

Absorbing new information, ideas, and philosophies that resonate with us takes time; and moving them into action and habits also takes time. As we evolve, layers reveal themselves as we are able to see, hear, and feel them. It's the rare person who would be exposed to a piece of life-changing information and then immediately assimilate and act on it. We can take in only so much at once, and how much we can take in, and how ready we are to do anything about it, varies from person to person. Sometimes I'll come into contact with an idea or some information, and I feel it gently nudge me in the ribs. It's like a nonconscious acknowledgment that the information is important to me. Weeks or months later, I'll be reading a book or having a conversation or watching a TED Talk, and I'm exposed to the information again, even if—or perhaps, especially if—it's presented a bit differently.

It's like the first nudge created a reference point in my mind that has since been growing and preparing itself for more. So the later exposure, say the TED Talk, will intrigue me, and I'm able to take in the information in a whole new way. And maybe at this point it's still theory—meaning, I'm still not doing anything to apply it to my way of thinking, doing, or being in the world. But I'm intrigued, philosophically. Then, a period of time later, I discover that learning to embody this intriguing philosophy is an ingredient that will alter my life experience in a profound way. Maybe that discovery happens as I'm working with how to help a client; or as I'm parenting a child and feeling as if we're constantly triggering each other; or as I open my mind and heart to a new understanding of what it means to be compassionate. Think of this book like these nudges; it's meant to be read and reread as various ideas attract you. Trust that what resonates with you will stay with you and will work its way through you; all you have to do is be open.

I want to honor that it's difficult to relax and embody all the uncertainty and ambiguity of messy personhood—and to own it all. This is the truth, and the truth is often inconvenient. We don't evolve how we honor our body, tend our mind, or live our spirit overnight. Deep, fundamental evolution takes time, as we challenge our existing patterns, physical (body) and psychological (mind). It's worth repeating: evolution in our lives typically happens with micromovements, not giant leaps or forced maneuvers. As always, some gentleness, patience, and kindness toward ourselves—in all of our beautiful, evolving messy personhood—goes a long way. Over time, our intention and efforts restructure us on cellular level. Literally. One layer at a time.

A Journey of Leaning In

You've likely noticed that I use the word *journey* quite a bit. And you likely picked up this book because you're interested in how to evolve your health, joy, and satisfaction with your life experience—how to express, live, and embody the most vibrant version of yourself. So I want to stress again, before we part ways, that this is most certainly a journey. What I've learned over the years, personally and professionally, is that "vibrant health" or "optimal health" doesn't mean "perfect health." It means being mindfully engaged with your health journey, BodyMindSpirit. It means we lean in, over time, to what best serves our wholeness.

BodyMindSpirit wholeness is about *so* much more than numbers: numbers on a scale, IQ tests, calorie numbers, SAT scores, numbers on blood tests. You're not a number. Health challenges, low spots, high spots, dis-ease, weight gain, weight loss, parenting issues, relationship issues, mindless relating, dimmer-switch-ology—are all *part* of your journey. They don't happen in spite of our health journey, or in the absence of it; they are it. The question isn't *"How much weight did you gain/lose?"* The questions are *"What did you learn? What can you evolve in your habits, choices, and environment?"* The question isn't *"What medication will alleviate the symptoms?"* The question is *"What foundational health challenges are causing the symptoms?"* The question isn't *"Why am I such a failure at relationships?"* The questions are *"What did I learn? How might I do it differently next time?"* Bumps and bruises along the path are all necessary grist for the mill. Our journey of leaning in is much more about asking good questions than about results. There is no "end result." It's a dance that you're engaged with, mindfully or not, throughout your life.

The best thing we can do is consistently, and with clear intentions, create a supportive environment for ourselves—within our body, in our minds, in our families, in our social groups, in our workplace, and in the communities that we choose to be part of. Celebrate what works, and be curious about what doesn't. Know that all conditions, within us and around us, are highly unstable; the only thing that's constant is impermanence—is change. Our life journey, and our health journey, are works in progress as we joyfully engage with our endless dance with impermanence.

An Idea Whose Time Has Come

We've covered a lot of ground together. Hopefully it's clear that there is no formula that we can all follow to create health and joy. The path that each of us takes toward the fullness of who we are is unique. We create the journey one little micromovement, one little habit, one little choice, and one little conversation at a time.

Our world is at a crucial tipping point—a fulcrum on which we'll tip toward peril or promise. The future rests in your hands—our future, and the future of our precious world. Einstein wrote, "The problems of the world will not be solved at the same level of thinking we were at when we created them." The cultural, political, economic, ecological, climatic, and other global issues that we currently face were created through prior ways of thinking. I therefore submit that the time for our personal evolution, and the turning up of our dimmer switch, is now.

We start with ourselves because we're worthy of a healthy and joyful life experience. We start with ourselves because our personal BodyMindSpirit journey feels good to us *and* helps us to sustain Love and stewardship for all that is. Health, joy, and personal evolution are both the journey and the fruit of our cherished life experience. Compassion, Love, and co-creation are our purpose, as embodied beings of OETU. We start with ourselves because our wholeness resonates out to the world of which we're a part.

Mind you, we don't necessarily need to set out to save the world. That can be a joyful and significant co-creation to take part in, and we can also be less all-in than that. The spark of sanity in a wild world happens in small ways at first. Maybe we set out to be curious about how other people are doing, and how our thoughts and actions might affect them. Maybe simple acts of compassion, toward loved ones and strangers, take root in our daily lives. Perhaps our contribution toward world sanity begins with the words we use with our child to discuss their behavior at school. Or possibly we become more mindful of our words on social media. This is how we begin to make the world a little healthier, a little more sane.

Indeed, our modern landscape is crying out for more health, balance, clarity, and Love. For more harmony and grace. For more space to hear the beating of our faithful human heart. There's nothing as powerful as an idea whose time has come; and the time has come for us to awaken to our innate health, joy, and interconnection—our innate well-being. And to live that with courage and passion. We'll never have a perfect world, and it would be impossible and dangerous to seek one. Aside from perfection being a myth, it would be challenging at best to reach consensus among the billions of members in our human family on what perfection looks, smells, tastes like. Yet evolution, from a place of integration and inclusivity—while honoring individuality and differentiation—is possible and needed. You are the one you've been waiting for.

My invitation to you is this: more often in your days, choose Love over fear, choose mindful over mindless, choose empowerment of others instead of power over others, choose honesty over lying, choose curiosity instead of toxic certainty, choose compassion over judgment. Choose to more joyfully inhabit your life, adjusting your dimmer switch so that your light shines and contributes to a more Loving and more sane world. Be kind and gentle with yourself, knowing that, while realizations are easy, the living of them can be a bit more tricky. The slightest "aha" moment, the tiniest opening of our hearts, the most subtle opening of the mind—these are major triumphs. For you, and for the evolution of our collective consciousness. This is exactly how evolution happens. We find something that works a little better for us, and we keep repeating it and expanding upon it. We live in our challenging times with a joyful heart, being the change that our precious world needs. This is how we create health and joy in a wild world.

GRATITUDE

It's hard to know how to fully express my deep well of gratitude for all of the people that contributed to this book's existence. As a first-time author, I learned what seasoned authors already know: there may be one name on the book's cover, but that one name would never make it to cover if it hadn't been for so many other people. I have no hope of identifying all of the influences on this book, but I'm going to do the best I can.

To Bob & Karen Boudreau, Claudia Herr, and my sweet mama Judy Warren: you are four people without whom I literally couldn't have given birth to this book. You're book doulas! Bob, not only did you insist that I get to work on my first book, but you and Karen also insisted on single-handedly removing some major obstacles on that path. Claudia, in addition to the wisdom and friendship that grew during our work together, thank you for your editorial strength and savvy, and for not running away screaming when I handed you a wordy, confusing manuscript almost twice as long as the finished book. Your patience and commitment are cape-worthy. Mom, you've supported and encouraged me for 53 years, and you're one of my dearest friends. To you four, thank you for your unshakeable faith in me and this book.

To my thoughtful and generous beta readers for their time and input. These friends helped this book become its best self: Monique Allen, Wendy Backlund, Claudia Doherty, Diane Hovenesian, Darren Roth, and Jim Masciarelli.

To my publicist Ashley Bernardi and her team at Nardi Media. Ashley, you're a joy to work and play with. Your excitement about this book got me through some dark days.

To the entire publishing team at Greenleaf for making the seemingly undo-able become do-able. I breathed a big sigh of relief when your seasoned team joined this project.

To the many other writers and writing professionals who have offered advice, input, and cheering on the long three-year road, including Andy Barzvi, Carol Bedrosian, Lucinda Blumenfeld, Wendy Capland, April Eberhardt, Kate Kaufmann, Mark Perna, Deborah Sosin, Lisa Tener, Angela Whitford, and the community at Grub Street.

To the Renegade Bookclub ladies, for being excited about this book, even when (especially when) I wasn't. Every month, you helped me keep going.

To Linda and Mark, for generously donating The Boathouse for many writing retreats on the coast of Maine, where inspiration and creativity come to me more easily. Thank you for the space to create, and for the love, camaraderie, and the Primo dates on my writing breaks.

In addition to those listed above, I'm grateful to the friends, clients, and colleagues who have challenged and inspired me along my own personal evolution, as a clinician/educator and as a person: Cora Alsante, Pamela Anderson, Christel Antonellis, Karl Backlund, Kim Barthel, Ashley Beaudoin, Trish Bertuzzi, Marie Carey, Dr. Kent Carter, Janet and Dennis Chandler, Michael Cinquino, Kelly Cotoia, Lauren and Steve Cummings, Dorothea Daniel, Tim Darter, Donna Davenport, Tracey Dodenhoff, Dr. Elaine Duffy, Rick Fritz, Dr. Albert Grazia, Corri Taylor, Dr. Cheryl Hardenbrook, Trish Hastry, Susan Hawkins, Martha Henry-MacDonald, Kim Huard-Michaud, Ron Imbriale, Drs. Wassim and Dawn Khoury, Dave and Michaela June, Lauren Killman, Steve Kramer, Mary LaRosa, Kristin Manning, Lauren Marciszyn, Donna Mitchell-Moniak, Seth Mleziva, Cheryl Moreland, the late Karl O'Connor, the playgroup ladies, Cathy Renda, Michelle Roccia, Dr. Anette Schippel, Gale Seaward,

Jeanne Sherlock, Dr. Lesley Shore, Dr. Linda Stoler, Sly, Sarah Terlaga, Bonnie Tragakis, Janine and Scott Wilkins, and Keith Wrightington.

To the teachers I've never met who wrote books that have educated, inspired, and empowered me—some that I've read many times over. As a voracious reader of nonfiction books, this list would be staggeringly long. The fact that we've never met doesn't change the fact that you've instructed my life journey and shaped my thoughts in some way, big or small. Thank you to writers of fabulous books.

To my clients, students, and Create Vibrant Health:BodyMindSpirit® community members: you inspire me, every day, to do work that serves others in the best way that I know how. I so enjoy our community and working together to transform the conversation around health and joy.

To the many colleagues, clients, friends, and family members who continued over the last three years to patiently ask, "So how's the book coming?" and offer words of excitement, support, and you-got-this. Every author I've every spoken to, seen interviews of, or read about has faced moments (days? weeks? months?) of despair and one small gesture of "You go, girl!" can make all the difference in a book actually making it through the eye of the needle, and on to its readers.

To the memory of Buz, with love.

To my late father, who educated and empowered me, in spite of himself: thank you for teaching me to think outside the box (what box?) and for instilling in me such a deep connection to our natural world.

To Leslie, Linda, Mark, and Pete: Thank you for your love, support, high fives, and fist bumps on this incredible journey of life. Sisterhood is a special bond, and I so scored in the brother-in-law department. Lucky me, all around.

To the four amazing people that I've had the honor and joy of parenting, step-parenting, and ex-step-parenting: Alex, Carolyn, Connor, and Jen. You are the four forever-loves of my life that I'm also lucky to call friends. We have a beautiful blended family and I love our life together. Thank you.

GLOSSARY

Aggression coping strategy: a communication coping strategy where we give ourselves permission to punish someone else for our pain and fear. It can include many "power-over" communication methods such as shaming, blaming, name-calling, humiliation, and toxic certainty.

Awareness: a slight shift in the way that we move through the world, where we move from life on automatic to life where we notice-the-not-usually-noticed. Our perception of our environment, of others, and of ourselves becomes softer and wider to include subtleties that we otherwise mentally dismiss. Awareness supports many aspects of empowered well-being. It is one of the Three Amigos and a foundational mindset in mindful relating.

Barrier: A self-created division that can be mental, physical, emotional, or spiritual. Barriers stop flow and connection.

Beliefs: the thoughts and opinions that we repeat over and over again until they become our personal dogma. They can be supportive or non-supportive to our well-being. Many of the beliefs we hold were programmed for us in our childhoods by authority figures such as parents, siblings, peers, coaches, and teachers.

BodyMindSpirit: a term that recognizes the human experience in its wholeness, and includes the aspect of emotion. The idea that we are physical, emotional, mental, and spiritual beings, and each aspect affects the well-being of the others.

Body Sass®: the homeo-dynamic state of balance, integration, and harmony in the body—being clinically well and feeling good in one's body. It's created and nurtured via intentional health-building habits and stewarding the BodyMindSpirit's ever-changing needs for balance.

Boundaries: self-created limits that can be physical, emotional, or mental and are critical for our health and well-being. Healthy boundaries exist when parties are clear with what is okay and not okay for each party. Boundaries support us in standing in who we are while also operating from a place of love and respect as we honor self and other. They are distinctly different than a barrier (see barrier). Boundaries are a foundational mindset in mindful relating.

Brain: the powerful physical organ that resides in the skull. The brain is the command center for the nervous system and controls body functions; it also interfaces with our mind. It's currently recognized as the most complex object known to humankind.

Challenge stress: (see Stress, challenge)

Chop wood and carry water: an ancient Buddhist teaching that points out that enlightenment is not an end-game. Before enlightenment, we chop wood and carry water; after enlightenment, we (still) chop wood and carry water. There's no before or after, nothing to achieve, and no big reveal. This teaching suggests that we bring all that we think, say, and do to our expansion of consciousness—to turning up our dimmer switch—as often as we can remember to do so.

Circle of concern: the vast array of life matters in our thoughts that we desire to have control over.

Circle of influence: the small number of life matters that lie within our circle of concern that we can impact. This circle is a small subset of our circle of concern (see circle of concern) and includes our attitude, our intention, and our perception.

Communication coping strategies: disconnection strategies that include aggression (attacking), shutting down (withdrawing), and conforming to please. These strategies are largely nonconscious and are focused on self-protection and/or winning, versus understanding and connection.

Compassion: the empathic desire to alleviate suffering; connects the *feeling* of empathy to *acts* of kindness, generosity, and understanding.

Conforming to please: a communication coping strategy, that's related to the withdrawal coping strategy, wherein someone internally disengages from true connection and interchange while appearing to be engaged. Occurs when we simply say and do what will be pleasing to the other in order to avoid discussion or confrontation.

Consciousness: includes our recognized mind functions, such as our five senses, as well as thought function, emotional processing, memory, intuition, and insight. It also includes our increasing awareness of the mystery of everything around us and within us, in addition to our being aware that we are aware of all that.

Conscious mind: (see mind, conscious)

Creator Mindset: a mindset that we own our life experience, and we understand that our health and joy are created and directed by the self. This mindset serves to empower us in expanding our potential for health, joy, and personal evolution.

Cue: the first step in the three-step mind-brain loop involved in habits. A cue is a trigger that creates craving and an increase of the neurotransmitter dopamine.

Curiosity: a state of wondering, and a desire to know more, that assists us in meeting the moment in a relaxed, open state. It's an approach—to learning, to people, to challenges, and to life—that opens the heart and mind. Curiosity supports many aspects of empowered well-being. It is one of the Three Amigos and a foundational mindset in mindful relating.

Dimmer switch: a metaphor that describes our ability to express varying degrees of our spirit aspect. The metaphor is founded on the belief that people all possess the same brilliance of spirit, while displaying a wide continuum of expression of that spiritual brilliance.

Dis-ease: a way of spelling the word "disease" that helps us remember that a diagnosis of "disease" is not a definitive prognosis of overall health. Instead of "disease" where the body is perceived as deceiving us, leaving us with a label of a sick person, dis-ease honors that the BodyMindSpirit can come out of balance, resulting in dis-ease in the integrity of our health.

Dogma: something that starts out as an idea gains traction, and people start to talk about the idea like it's a 100 percent truth that can't be argued. The inherent belief is that this way is the only right way, the inarguable truth. In common vernacular, dogma is often related to religion; but dogma can be created in any structure of ideals, including science and medicine.

Dopamine: a neurotransmitter released when we anticipate *or* experience pleasure. It is also involved in movement, memory, and focus.

Emotional intelligence: our ability to be aware of, navigate, and express emotions. It encompasses intrapersonal (within ourselves) and interpersonal (between us and someone else) emotional savvy. It exists along a continuum.

Emotions: powerful and important currents of specific Energies that each have their own frequency, character, movement, and use. They're an internal navigation tool that's first felt in the body, and then processed with our mind.

Energy-with-a-capital-E: the organizing Energy of the universe. All is created from this Energy, which can be neither created nor destroyed. It forms and instructs everything from thoughts to stones, from beetles to radio waves, from plankton to human tissue.

Environment: the external conditions and resources surrounding an organism, along with all physical, emotional, mental, and spiritual stimuli that influence the organism. An organism can be as small as a cell (or smaller) and as large as planet Earth (or larger).

Food Sass®: whole, organic, nutrient-dense foods that are as close to their original state as possible. These foods are typically found at farm stands or around the perimeter of the market and contain a combination of clean protein, healthy fats, and complex carbohydrates. The foods provide phytochemicals, vitamins, and minerals in their original state and contribute to a plant-slant food lifestyle that is enjoyable and full of variety.

Forgiveness: an ongoing, conscious decision made by our whole selves to release our feelings of resentment or vengeance. It allows us to release the past, heal, and live more fully in the present.

Generosity: the quality of deeply considering the other-than-self such as other people, animals, the environment, the planet. Generosity is also acting on that consideration with Love. Generosity can take many forms, including time, presence, money, heart, and spirit.

Gratitude: being intentionally thankful for what feels good to us in our life experience, which encourages us to feel grateful, abundant, and generous a little more regularly. We start to appreciate more and more of our life experience in whatever form that takes. Gratitude leads to increased feelings of connection, joy, and well-being.

Habit: an action, routine, thought, or behavior that we perform regularly and is often automatic. It's estimated that 40 to 50 percent of our actions are run by habits.

Health: balance, integration, and ease—overall well-being—in body, emotions, mind, and spirit. Whole-person health is created from within and tended on an ongoing basis.

Holding space: the generous act of being with a person while consciously embodying awareness, presence, nonjudgment, and love. When holding space, we compassionately witness another's emotional state, while staying grounded in our Being.

Humility: a tendency to focus outward from a base of compassion, generosity, gratitude, and kindness. Humble folks have a real interest in others and in the world at large. A humble person tends to be self-aware, including having a dispassionate awareness of their limitations.

Intention: how we direct our consciousness toward manifesting what we'd like to create, achieve, or have. Intention directs Energy, guiding manifestation of our desires. Intention is a foundational mindset of mindful relating.

Joy: a state of being that is best described as a mix of delight, contentment, connection, and harmony. It often includes awe. It arises from the heart and spirit and is not affected or caused by outside circumstances. Joy, in a very real way, is experiencing exactly what's happening, minus our opinion of it.

Justification: a me-first communication tactic where we communicate to ourselves and others that we had no choice but to say or do the unkind, unsupportive, or hurtful thing that we previously said or did. We lean on excuses to justify and explain away our weak, unkind, or inconsiderate words and behavior.

Kindness: doing or communicating something that we perceive and hope will benefit another(s) without expecting anything in return. It's rooted in empathy and acceptance, and comes from our integrity and our heart. Kindness has its roots in personal ethics and is a heartfelt concern for others and ourselves.

Love: the endless and pervading vibration of the Organizing Energy of the Universe that reveals itself to us in an endless myriad of ways such as the intelligence of the natural world, kindness, generosity, compassion, peace, intimacy, connection, mindful relating, joy, and empathy.

Me-first relating: relating style focused on the self—how can I most easily defend myself and get my way? Me-first relating is the opposite of we-first relating or mindful relating.

Meditation: a heightened state of awareness in the moment, where someone continually and without judgment brings the mind back to a point of focus (often the breath).

Messy personhood: the part of the mind that is responsible for our sense of being a separate personal identity who uniquely strives and suffers. We feel separate from everything around us and therefore feel the need to protect what's "ours." Since we're deeply interconnected with all of the beings and life around us, this results in us feeling stressed, confused, emotionally polarized, less than, more than, depressed, power hungry, victimized, anxious, lonely, and messy. Similar to the psychology term "ego."

Micromovements: tiny habits—in the form of actions and thoughts—that we consistently repeat to move toward our goals and desires. Setting an alarm clock at night is a micromovement of the larger habit of being punctual to work in the morning.

Mind: the seat of our human-ness. It includes the felt sense of self, thought, our ability to be aware of the world and of our experiences, memory, as well as faculties like intuition. There are aspects of mind that we can loosely associate with areas of the brain, as the brain can act as a receptor for mind activity. The mind does not *live* anywhere, as it's a nonphysical aspect of being human.

Mind, conscious: the part of our psyche that includes direct awareness, where we experience ourselves and our environment directly through sensory experience, such as sight, sound, taste, hearing, touch, and mental activity.

Mind, nonconscious: the aspect of mind that functions on autopilot (seat of our habits and beliefs), including our mental storage center and all mental activity that is not in our awareness.

Mind-brain, or **mind-brain system:** a term used in contexts where we're unclear on what is associated with mind versus brain. It's often difficult to separate mind function from brain function, as they're deeply interdependent.

Mindful relating: also known as we-first relating, where all parties involved focus on strengthening connection, one of our most basic needs. Mindful relating is co-creation of connection and understanding, while exercising compassion and utilizing the Ten Healing Practices.

Mindfulness: open, active attention to the present moment, with an awareness that the present moment simply *is*. It's a conscious, purposeful way of tuning in to what's happening right now, within us and around us, without judgment. Mindfulness supports many aspects of empowered well-being, is one of the Three Amigos, and is also a foundational mindset in mindful relating.

A Moment: when we respond to a trigger in our environment in a way that wakes us up to a wider perspective in our world-view. The trigger—words, actions, observations, interactions—sparks a realization that our perspective is only one way of seeing things, and that there are many different ways of viewing the same thing.

Nonconscious mind: (see mind, nonconscious)

OETU: an intentionally unaffiliated acronym for the Organizing Energy of the Universe; what some folks call God, Allah, Almighty, Jehovah, Father, Brahma, Christ, Gaia, or another name; a Divine energy that instructs all that is.

Observer, inner: a concept that assists us in observering our mind. This observation is devoid of emotions, judgment, and criticism, while we watch and reflect upon exactly what is observed, like a mirror.

Open heart: a heart that compassionately honors the messy personhood of others—along with our own—with a willingness to be curious and vulnerable. It allows us to have necessary boundaries without constructing barriers; a foundational mindset of mindful relating.

Pain: an uncomfortable mental or physical response to something that happens in the moment. Pain can lead to suffering.

Personal responsibility: the ability to respond to our environment through conscious choice and know that other people are not responsible for the personal suffering in our mind. It lies at the very heart of empowered Body-MindSpirit well-being and means that we hold ourselves accountable for what we think, say, and do. One of the Three Pillars that are foundational to our empowered well-being.

Perspective: how we see or interpret the world around us.

The Present: now, this moment, the only time that is in existence.

Projection: a me-first communication tactic where we hurl what we don't like about ourselves onto the people and world around us, so that we can rail against it while still being defended. Projection occurs when we attribute to others something that's true for ourselves. For instance, we accuse someone of being controlling when we are, in fact, struggling with our desire for control.

Psychological stress: (see Stress, psychological)

Psychological time: a mind-created construct where we move outside of the reality of clock time and combine the passage of time with emotions and psychological fear. Is a significant contributor to psychological stress and anxiety.

Relaxation response: a biochemical and physiological result of our parasympathetic nervous system being activated. It promotes balance—in the moment and cumulatively over time—within our nervous system and our entire body by offsetting the stress response activated by our sympathetic nervous system.

Resistance: our internal railing against what *is*, when we're wanting the present moment to be different than it is. It creates emotional turbulence and stress turbulence within our psyche and is the cause of most of our suffering.

Reverence: a deep humility-inspiring awe for all that is; an attitude of honoring life in all its manifestations.

Reward: the third step in the three-step loop involved in habits. Reward is how our brain decides if the feedback loop feels beneficial to us or not. Does the Routine in step two bring about the feelings of pleasure that we've learned to expect?

Routine: the second step in the three-step habit loop. An activity, emotion, or behavior that can be replaced as long as it delivers feelings of satisfaction or Reward, via dopamine.

Self-care: identifying individual needs for BodyMindSpirit well-being and taking steps to meet them, on a daily basis, acting from a place of support and love. Self-care is provided for you, by you and is one of the Three Pillars that are foundational to empowered well-being.

Self-referencing: a me-first communication tactic where we override the attempts of others to be seen and heard by bringing the conversation back to our experiences, our wants, our needs.

Self-worth: a sense of one's own intrinsic value or worth as a person. It is confidence in our unique expression of personhood and an unshakeable faith in ourselves. Self-worth is one of the Three Pillars that are foundational to our empowered well-being.

Sensitives: people who have more depth of processing, are more easily over-stimulated, are more sensitive to subtleties in our environment, and/or feel emotions more strongly than the majority of people.

Stress: our perception of events, circumstances, and thoughts as being demanding or adverse.

Stress, challenge: when we perceive and respond to challenging stimuli as opportunities to help us learn, grow, and become stronger.

Stress, psychological: when we perceive and react to challenging stimuli as being overwhelming and insurmountable, leaving us to feel threatened, help-less, and in a victim state. We often mentally dwell on these stimuli, imagining worst-case scenarios, without taking real action to respond to the challenge.

Stress, survival: when our ability to correctly perceive and respond to per-ceived threats via fight, flight, or freeze can be life-saving.

Stress management: habits and tactics that we can practice in our everyday lives to offset the accumulation of mental angst and stress hormones, and to help us to build stress resilience. Most of these tactics invoke the relaxation response, which biochemically opposes the stress response.

Stress resilience: our ability to withstand and adapt to what we perceive as stressors and adverse events. Becomes stronger and more deeply ingrained as we practice stress management tactics and work to positively evolve our relationship with our mind and emotions.

Suffering: a mental exacerbation of pain where we continually focus on, relive, or magnify prior or current pain.

Surrender: the antidote to resistance, the cause of the vast majority of our suffering. Surrender is relinquishing our attachment to the outcome. It's about yielding to the flow of life in this moment, recognizing what IS. An unconditional acceptance of the present moment does not exclude the possibility of future damage control, taking action, initiating change, pursuing goals, and the like.

Survival stress: (see Stress, survival)

Symptom: a messenger that communicates internal imbalance from body to mind, allowing our mind to register that there's a problem to be addressed.

The Ten Healing Practices: strategies that support our personal evolution toward a more receptive, curious, and powerful mind: mindfulness, gratitude, humor, simplicity, generosity, perspective, meditation, humility, forgiveness, and the present. The Ten Healing Practices move us from using the mind as a barrier to using the mind as a bridge, creating health, joy, and personal evolution.

The Three Amigos: the natural, innate human states of awareness, curiosity, and mindfulness.

Toxic certainty: a me-first communication tactic where we express opinions as facts. When we're so sure that we're right, that we have little ability to hear anything else. Often accompanied by feelings of intellectual or emotional superiority and/or contempt for others, either privately or verbally.

Trauma, psychological: damage to the psyche as a result of any type of mind-brain or physical stimulus that, in its intensity, sends a person into dissociation without the ability to come fully back into themselves.

Victim Mindset: a mindset that our life experience happens outside of us and "at" us, dictating that our health and joy are created and directed by outside influences. This mindset serves to dilute our vast potential, as we then continually look for answers outside of ourselves to liberate us from our discomfort, our dissatisfaction, and our pain.

We-first relating: a relating style that focuses on the relationship at hand, instead of on ourselves. It encompasses a relational paradigm shift that has curiosity at its heart. We-first relating is the opposite of me-first relating. Also called mindful relating.

Willpower: our ability to resist immediate temptations or desires that are not in support of our long-term goals. Is a quickly exhaustible and exhausting resource that is best reserved for supporting habit change, as opposed to a means to an end in and of itself. Also known as self-control or self-discipline.

Withdrawal coping strategy: a communication coping strategy in which a person withdraws from active interchange in communication, quite literally disconnecting and shutting down. Withdrawal is the opposite of the aggression coping strategy.

ABOUT THE AUTHOR

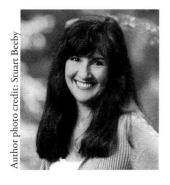

Laurie Warren, MSN, Vibrant Living Advocate is the founder of Create Vibrant Health: BodyMindSpirit®, through which she joyfully educates and inspires others to create empowered well-being.

Warren runs a holistic health and healing practice, employing two decades of study in science, functional medicine, and psychology for her clients' better health. A sought-after speaker, her expertise is also regularly featured in the media, including recent interviews on CNN's *Headline News* and Washington DC's Fox5 News and WBUR.

In her corporate consulting work, Warren blends experience from an early twelve-year business career in high tech with her expertise in physical and mental well-being to help companies build progressive wellness cultures. One of her clients, the northeast recruiting firm WinterWyman, won a Boston's Healthiest Companies award in 2014 as a result of their partnership with her.

Laurie lives in the Greater Boston area and enjoys the life she gets to share with her four children and her two grandchildren. In her free time, she spends time in the great outdoors.